Child Development

BYWORD BOOKS™

We strongly discourage self-medication. The reader is urged to read the printed instructions of drug companies as well as consult a physician before using any of the drugs mentioned in this book because new side-effects are recognized and dosage schedules are being constantly revised. It is possible that errors might have crept in despite our best efforts.

First published 2007
Reprinted 2008, 2010, 2011

10 9 8 7 6 5 4 3 2 1

ISBN 81-8193-031-2
ISBN 978-81-8193-031-6

Published by
Byword Books Private Limited
Virat Bhavan, Mukherjee Nagar Commercial Complex, Delhi 110009
email: bywordbooks@gmail.com
website: www.bywordbooks.in

Printed at Manipal Press Ltd, India

DoctorNDTV Team

Parul Chopra
Yatish Jain
Surjeet Bisht
Neha Vij
Pankaj Matta

Dr Anurag Krishna
Dr Anuj Sharma
Dr Nazli Siddiqui
Dr Shirish Kumar
Dr Samiran Nundy

Consulting Editor

Dr S. Anandalakshmy
Consultant in Child Development and Education, Chennai

Experts

Dr Renu Kishore
Reader, Department of Psychology, University of Delhi, Delhi

Dr Jitendra Nagpal
Senior Consultant Psychiatrist, Vidyasagar Institute of Mental Health and Neurosciences, New Delhi

Dr Samir Parikh
Consultant Psychiatrist and Chief, Department of Mental Health and Behavioural Sciences, Max Healthcare, New Delhi

Dr Veena Kalra
Paediatric Neurologist, All India Institute of Medical Sciences, New Delhi

Ms Kavita Sharma
Principal, Hindu College, University of Delhi, Delhi

Dr Nipun Kashyap
Developmental Paediatrician, Indraprastha Apollo Hospitals, New Delhi

Dr Ajit Harisinghani
Speech Therapist, Speech Foundation, Pune

Dr Mel Levine
Director, Clinical Center for the Study of Development and Learning
University of North Carolina, USA

Ms Shyama Chona
Principal, Delhi Public School, R.K. Puram, New Delhi

Dr Swati Bhave
Adolescent Specialist, Max Healthcare, New Delhi

Ms Jyoti Bose
Principal, Spingdales School, New Delhi

Preface

In April 2000 during a convivial Sunday lunch at the Roys we were discussing how information on health was sadly out of the reach of most people living in India. Unlike the situation in western countries, especially in the USA, where important newspapers such as the *New York Times* had a special and authoritative section devoted to health every Tuesday, no such information was accessible in India. The newspapers and major television channels at that time carried few health stories and consequently anyone who was sick had to rely on a paternalistic doctor for all his or her health information. The busy doctor was usually reluctant to answer a patient's queries in detail and was likely to be irritated by the 'troublesome' patient who asked for more information. The patient was also hesitant to ask too many questions, as this would waste the doctor's time.

Two events occurred which changed the doctor-patient relationship in this country. The first was the passage of the Consumer Protection Act, which brought the medical profession under its purview in 1995. This allowed patients to take doctors to court for what they or their relatives perceived to be malpractice. The dissatisfaction with medical care was often due to a lack of communication between the doctor and the patient or due to the unrealistic expectations of the patient. Outright malpractice was rare as reflected by the very few judgments given against doctors.

The second event was the arrival of health websites on the internet. These began appearing in large numbers, most of them with obviously commercial intent and blatantly promoted hospitals, doctors or drugs. It was not possible to distinguish whether or not the information they provided was reliable. Nevertheless, these websites became immensely popular and, in the year 2000, it was estimated that 40% of American households were accessing the net for health information. Unfortunately, these websites targeted largely a western audience and carried little information of relevance to Indian patients because our diseases, technology available and social conditions were so different.

At that lunch we decided to start a not-for-profit health website in India which would cater exclusively to Indians providing them reliable information which was appropriate to their social and economic circumstances and would be of an 'international' quality. All of the information provided would be completely free.

We first sent emails to a hundred or so of our friends and acquaintances, who were leaders in medicine in this country and abroad, inviting them to join our site called DoctorNDTV. We explained to them that their responsibilities would include writing short articles on common and rare Indian diseases in a standardized question–answer format, vetting the material that our in-house staff produced and answering queries that had been emailed to us. All of this they were expected to do without any remuneration. Surprisingly, more than ninety per cent of these experts agreed to join.

We recruited medical colleagues – Dr Anuj Sharma, a web-savvy clinical microbiologist; Dr Anurag Krishna, a paediatric surgeon; Dr Shirish Kumar, a clinical haematologist; and Dr Nazli Siddiqui, a family physician – as well as bright young people to work on content – Pooja Gupta, Vibha Baluja, Jaieta Nag, Parul Chopra, Neha Vij and Surjeet Bisht – and technical staff – Sankalp Singh, Yugant Khanna and Pankaj Matta. Of these Parul, Neha and Surjeet are still with us while the others have moved on.

DoctorNDTV.com was launched in November 2000 and in its first year attracted about 5000 page-views a month and about 10 queries a day (all of which were answered within 72 hours). It is now the leading Indian health website for the general public and attracts over 4 million page-views a month and has 290 experts from all over the world who answer about 120 queries a day (the answer rate at present is about 90% – overwhelmed as we are by the numbers). From these we archive daily about 5–7 of the most useful and interesting questions and answers so that they are more easily accessible.

To make these archived Q&As available (and affordable, thanks to a subsidy from NDTV) to a wider public – those without computers or those on the move – we thought we would organize Q&As into printed books on individual topics. After analysing the kind of questions we are sent we found that the most frequently asked ones have been on sex, pregnancy and child development; so we have started the series with books on these three subjects.

After reading the DoctorNDTV books we hope that the next time you visit your doctor you will be able to better understand what the doctor says, and ask the most relevant questions regarding what's the matter of concern with you, and how and when things might improve.

SAMIRAN NUNDY
Editor-in-Chief
DoctorNDTV.com

May 2007

Introduction

All parents tend to have occasional doubts about whether their children are developing normally and whether they, as parents, are doing the right thing for them. Sometimes, parents may feel that they need the advice of an expert whom they can consult, while their own identity remains confidential. The assurance of anonymity seems to help them to unburden themselves and to be candid. The free service of the NDTV panel of doctors and counsellors opens up the possibility for parents to get answers to their questions.

As the people answering these questions, we try and reconstruct the home or school situation - which the letters mention only briefly - and to read between the lines. For many of us, it is more challenging than a personal, face-to-face consultation, where we could have read the body language and caught the nuance as well. Perhaps, we make mistakes, unwittingly, in our interpretation of a question. At times, the response we give may not satisfy a parent, who wants an instant solution to a problem. In most cases, our replies only indicate a direction the parent can take. For us, the lack of feedback from those we have advised, is a frustration, but we keep going. The hope, that our voice is listened to and may help someone, sustains our work.

This selection of questions that we receive reflects the common issues of childhood and parenting in our society. Our optimism leads us to believe that the answers from the team of psychologists may provide guidance to a wide cross-section of families in this country and elsewhere.

S. ANANDALAKSHMY
Consulting Editor

Contents

List of questions

Infants and toddlers (birth to 3 years)

School issues

Sleep concerns

Preschoolers (3 to 5 years)

Difficult children

Miscellaneous

6 to 9 year olds

School issues

Disciplining children

Sex education

Miscellaneous

Adolescents

School issues

Behaviour/habits

Appendix

Infants and toddlers (birth to 3 years)

- Markers of growth
- Social behaviour
- Sibling rivalry
- Thumb-sucking
- Toys for young children

- Behaviour
- Fussy eaters
- School issues
- Sleep concerns

Markers of growth

Watching a baby grow is a fascinating and unique experience for the parents. A child's growth is a complex and continuous process. A child is usually able to do different things at certain stages. These can be termed as *markers of growth*. It is important to realize that no two children grow at the same rate. At the ages noted for different activities, the child should be observed for some time. The child may develop more slowly in certain areas than other children of the same age while his other activities may be ahead of other children.

Everything is a new and exciting experience for a newborn baby. She is always absorbing information through her five senses - sight, sound, smell, touch and taste. Human beings never stop learning, but the rate at which babies learn is much faster than that of an adult. The baby's emotions and intellect are developing during the first weeks of life, just as rapidly as size, weight and coordination. There are no hard and fast rules. These markers are not rigid or fixed. Each child is a unique individual. She follows her own individual pattern for growth. There are early developers and late developers. These are individual patterns and as any child specialist will tell you *not* a cause for concern. However, a check-up by a paediatrician is needed to rule out any medical complication and put the parents at ease. 'She' is used to denote both boy and girl.

Infants and toddlers (birth to up to 3 years)

Rapid screening for growth delay
2 months - social smile
4 months - holding neck
8 months - sitting without support
12 months - standing, can spot small moving objects

Birth to 8 weeks (2 months)

What the baby understands in the first three months
Focusing on objects and distinguishing voices.

The newborn baby
- Can focus on your face and recognize it
- Can also distinguish your voice.

Four weeks
- Lies on the back with head turned to one side
- Sudden noise startles the baby making the body stiff

- The fists are clenched
- May grasp an object that touches her palm
- Will start recognizing you as a source of comfort and stop crying when you pick her up.

Eight weeks

- Will focus on a brightly coloured object held above her head
- Then follow it with her gaze as you move it from side to side.

Physical and motor-skill markers

- Closure of the soft spot at the back of the head
- Baby appears to dance or step when placed upright on solid surface
- Less head lag
- When on stomach, the baby is able to lift head to almost 45 degrees
- Less flexing of the arms and legs while on stomach.

Sensory and cognitive markers

- Head turns from side-to-side with sound close to the ear
- Begins to look at close objects
- Cries differently when in pain or hunger
- Vocal response to familiar voices
- Smiles
- Will smile back at you
- Eyes will be able to follow a moving toy.

Three months to six months

Three months

- Will immediately look at a toy held in front of the eyes
- Will smile when you speak and squeal and gurgle with pleasure
- Will show obvious signs of curiosity and interest.

Four months

Physical and motor-skill markers

- Shows a slowing of weight gain to approximately 20 grams per day
- Demonstrates the fading of the infant reflexes
- Has almost no head lag while in a sitting position
- Able to sit up straight if propped
- Raises head to 90 degrees when placed on stomach
- Able to roll from front to back
- Tries to reach objects with hands
- Plays with rattle when it is placed in the hands, but will not be able to pick it up if dropped

- Able to grasp rattle with both hands
- Able to place objects in mouth.

Sensory and cognitive markers

- Has well-established close vision
- Begins to have eye–hand coordination
- Able to laugh out loud
- Demands attention by fussing
- Recognizes parent's voice or touch
- Will react in an excited manner at feeding time
- Will laugh and chuckle when played with
- Will turn its head towards any sound.

Six months

Physical and motor-skill markers

- Should have doubled birth weight by 4 months, and it is a matter of concern if it has not happened by 6 months
- Able to lift chest and head while on stomach, bearing the weight on hands (often occurs by 4 months)
- Able to sit in a high chair with a straight back
- Beginning of teething
- Increased drooling
- Able to bear almost all weight when supported in a standing position
- Able to roll from back to stomach
- Able to hold her own bottle for short periods
- Able to pick up a dropped object.

Sensory and cognitive markers

- Can locate sounds not made directly at the ear level
- Prefers more complex sound stimulation
- Starts to imitate sounds
- Sounds resemble one-syllable words
- Makes sounds to mirror and toys. The baby will also be fascinated by mirror as she can see herself.
- Begins to fear strangers
- Recognizes parents
- Begins to imitate actions
- The baby will be able to differentiate between different kinds of food and develop dietary preferences.

Seven months to ten months

Seven months

- Will start understanding simple words and playing.

Eight months

- Will know its name and will understand the concept of 'no'
- Will try to attract your attention by making little sounds.

Nine months

Physical and motor-skill markers

- Gains weight at a slower rate – approximately 15 grams per day
- Increases in length by 1.5 cm per month
- Bowel and bladder systems become more regulated
- Is able to protect self from falling
- Is able to crawl
- Remains sitting for prolonged periods
- Pulls self to standing position
- Can grasp with thumb and index finger
- Can feed self if allowed to do so
- Throws or shakes objects.

Sensory and cognitive markers

- Develops depth perception
- Achieves 'object constancy' – the understanding that objects continue to exist even when not seen
- Responds to simple commands
- Responds to name
- Imitates speech sounds
- May be afraid of being left alone
- Plays interactive games
- Will exhibit a will of her own
- Will display an interest in toys and games.

Ten months

- Will be able to clap her hands and wave goodbye
- Will also show that she understands a few words and very short, simple statements.

Eleven months to fifteen months

Eleven months

- Will enjoy games and dropping things
- Will be fascinated by sound and will want to shake and bang objects.

Twelve months

Physical and motor-skill markers

- Triples the birth weight
- Grows to a height of 50% over birth length
- Has a head circumference equal to that of the chest
- Has 6–8 teeth
- Stands and walks with help or alone
- Sits down without help
- Can bang two blocks together
- Turns through pages of a book by flipping many at a time
- Has a precise pincer grasp.

Sensory and cognitive markers

- Follows a fast-moving object
- Has control over response to sounds
- Comprehends several words
- Can say mamma, papa, and at least 1–2 other words
- Comprehends simple commands
- Points to objects with index finger
- Waves bye
- Will derive great pleasure in making you laugh and will repeatedly do things that amuse you
- Will enjoy looking at books
- Will have learned a few simple words.

Fifteen months

- Will want to brush her own hair
- Will understand the meaning of kissing
- May not understand individual words, but will be able to comprehend a few complex sentences.

Eighteen months to twenty-one months

Eighteen months

Physical and motor-skill markers

- Has a closed anterior fontanelle (soft spot on the front of the head)
- Grows at a slower rate and has less of an appetite compared to previous months
- Runs with a lack of coordination and falls frequently
- Jumps in place
- Is able to get onto chairs without assistance
- Walks up stairs while holding on with one hand
- Can build a tower of 2–3 blocks

- Can use a spoon and cup with help
- Imitates scribbling
- Can turn 2–3 pages of a book at a time.

Sensory and cognitive markers

- Shows affection
- Listens to a story or looks at pictures
- Can say 10 or more words when asked
- Identifies parts of the body
- Understands and is able to point to and identify common objects such as dog, cow, ball, etc.
- Frequently imitates
- Feeds self
- If you ask her to fetch something, she will.

Twenty-one months

- Will understand and obey simple requests
- Will come to you and draw your attention towards things that interest her
- Will love scribbling with a pencil.

The third year

This is the stage when your child's favourite word is 'why'. The child will be inquisitive about several objects. She will now learn to establish links between different things. The child's sense of creativity and imagination will be awakened. The child will learn to think ahead and to plan.

Physical and motor-skill markers

- Should have the first 16 teeth (the actual number could vary widely)
- Runs with better coordination, while the stance may remain wide
- Kicks ball without losing balance
- Can build a tower of 6–7 cubes
- Browses through a book one page at a time
- Able to turn a door knob
- Picks up objects while standing, without losing balance.

Sensory and cognitive markers

- Vision fully developed
- Vocabulary increased to about 50–300 words
- Can organize phrases of 2–3 words
- Able to communicate needs such as thirst and hunger
- Increased attention span

- Able to clothe self in simple clothes; better at removing clothes than putting them on
- Becomes quite self-sufficient and can amuse herself
- Will be happy playing by herself
- Will know the names of familiar objects and how to use them.

Two years, three months
- Will develop a sense of self
- Knows who she is and can say her name
- Will become more assertive about what she wants
- Will impose her will against yours
- Will try to build houses and castles with toy bricks

Two years, six months
- Will know both, her first name and her surname
- Will enjoy lending you a hand with simple chores
- Will be able to draw vertical and horizontal lines.

Two years, nine months
- Will know the difference between boys and girls
- Will be able to learn nursery rhymes and repeat them
- Will ask questions and begin to understand numbers
- Will try to draw a circle, but will not succeed without help.

Social behaviour

The social development of the child is as important as her physical and intellectual development. The child must be able to communicate and interact with other people. Every baby has a unique personality waiting to be developed. Watching the baby grow and unfold its individual persona is a unique experience. She has her own likes and dislikes. As the baby learns to express herself better, her personality gets revealed to us. The development of a baby from a passive creature to a social being is a very fascinating process.

Baby's behaviour during the first year

At three months

The baby will display a liking for company and human contact. She will express her displeasure by crying when she is ignored or left alone. She will express pleasure when others are around by smiling, kicking her legs or waving her arms. She will turn around and look when people are speaking and smile when you speak to her. She will recognize familiar faces and react towards strangers by crying or turning away.

Four to six months

The baby will focus on faces and follow a person with her eyes when he walks away. She will lift her hands in a gesture indicating that you should pick her up. She will laugh when you pay attention to her and play with her. Your baby will be able to understand that you are angry. She will smile at familiar people and show visible signs of fear towards strangers. At six months, your baby will become more interactive, pulling the hair of the person holding her, rubbing noses with them or patting their faces.

Seven to twelve months

Your baby will begin to imitate speech sounds and gestures. She will desist from whatever she is doing when you say 'no'. She will become more clingy at this stage and express fear and dislike of strangers by rushing to your side or crying.

Baby's behaviour during the second year

Most of the toddler's actions are aimed at attracting your attention. Thus, she may try speaking to you, crying, hitting you or annoying you. She is not particular whether the attention is positive or negative as long as she can catch your eye. Once you respond to her, she will smile or laugh at you. Your baby will have frequent mood swings, between extreme displays of affection and anger. The child will become more participative in play and this is a good opportunity to teach her to share.

A naughty child

A naughty child is one who knows the difference between right and wrong, but lacks the maturity to exert self-control and do the right thing. You have to be very patient with naughty children. Initially, you should try to have a sympathetic approach and speak to them frequently. If this fails, restricting or withdrawing privileges is a much more effective way.

A disobedient child

A disobedient child is to be dealt with great patience. Physical punishment is likely to lead to aggression. Explain to the child that her activities are not acceptable and suggest how she should behave. (*See also* page 100)

A shy and timid child

Some children are naturally shy. They do not speak much and keep to themselves. Other children are chatterboxes at home. However, when they are introduced into a new situation or to new people, they seem to withdraw into a shell. Such children cannot be thrust into a new situation. You have to give them time to adjust. Do not try to force them to join in immediately. Encourage them to socialize when they feel comfortable.

An aggressive child

Aggression in a child is usually the result of parental neglect, their absence or too much or too little discipline. Aggressive children are usually bullies, they physically and verbally attack children much smaller than them. The best way to deal with them is to clearly demonstrate disapproval and to praise good behaviour. (*See also* page 100)

Sibling rivalry

One of the most traumatic events in your child's life can be the arrival of a new baby. For a toddler, adapting to a new baby in the house can be a very stressful experience.

Why does it happen?

Between the ages of 18 months and 3-and-a-half years, a child is just beginning to establish her individual identity by collecting bits and pieces of information about herself. During this time she is also beginning to realize that she is a separate individual from her parents. This knowledge makes her feel insecure and vulnerable and she becomes very possessive about her own things. So, the arrival of a sibling at this stage can seem to be exceptionally threatening. When someone invades our space, it is normal for us to react with some concern. This is exactly what the arrival of a new baby makes your toddler feel. She will feel displaced and threatened by the attention and physical contact the newborn gets from her mother. Her parents seem to no longer belong exclusively to her; moreover she loses the role of the baby of the family.

What about jealous reactions?

Any jealous reactions may be dormant until the new baby is old enough to steal the attention of people. At first there may not be much rivalry. Children younger than 20 months actually tolerate a newborn intruder much better than those over 2 years of age, because they are not aware of being displaced. Jealous reactions seem more intense in first-born children than in others, probably because they have the most to lose. They might revert to increased thumb-sucking, more than the usual amount of babyish chatter, cranky demanding behaviour, or excessive clinging.

How to deal with them?

You may not be able to totally eliminate possessiveness or jealousy. Psychologists believe that coping with these emotions helps a child mature. Parents can only diffuse the intensity of these emotions through proper handling.

Before the baby comes

Even if your toddler is not saying much and you are not really sure what she understands, it is important to fill her in. Knowing what to expect will ease the transition once the baby actually arrives. About 3 or 4 months before the baby is due, it would be good to tell your child as simply and truthfully as possible about the new birth. Describe the changes that will take place in your household once the baby arrives. Assure her that none of the changes will affect her, that she will continue to be loved as before.

Let your child help

Although they may not always seem so, toddlers generally are interested in their new brothers or sisters. Take advantage of that curiosity by letting your child participate in the baby's care. It would be wise not to leave the baby alone with her just yet. Even a simple chitchat about what you are doing when bathing the baby or cleaning him, would help your older child feel involved. Emphasize your toddler's big-sister status by putting her in charge of telling you if she hears the baby cry.

According to experts, at around one month of age, infants begin to recognize their sibling, which may help a child accept the little newcomer. Encourage your toddler to sing and talk to the baby, and see how the baby's face lights up.

Provide your valuable time

Rather than scolding her for any feelings of jealousy, acknowledge her feelings so she knows you understand her point of view. Take some time each day to do something just with her, even if it is only for a few minutes. If your baby goes to sleep earlier than your older child, designate an hour or two as 'big child time'.

What needs to be done?

Young children who feel jealous commonly act on these feelings. Do not be surprised if your toddler hits or throws something at her new sibling. This is normal though not easy to witness. When you are alone with her, encourage her to express her feelings. It is necessary to intervene immediately if she is aggressive, but not to physically punish or humiliate her.

Toddlers often regress when a new baby comes into the house. Regressing in behaviour and speech is one way of coping. You may suddenly see your child talking like a baby. Children aren't too sophisticated in asking what they really need. When they need attention, they often represent this in their behaviour. Parents should recognize this need for attention. They should respond to it somewhat, but also try to encourage more age-appropriate behaviour through praise and attention when the child acts her age.

Is it necessary to give it time?

Do not expect your older child to be happy about the arrival of a baby sister or brother. Just give your toddler as much love, undivided attention and understanding as it takes to make it through the first few months. Make sure your expectations of your toddler do not suddenly exceed reasonable levels. You cannot expect her to grow up suddenly because an infant has arrived. The contrast between her abilities and the helplessness of a new baby puts a lot of pressure on her to abandon her immaturity. If she reverts to babyish behaviour, additional hugs and kisses are more likely to improve the situation than reprimands.

Thumb-sucking

A habit is a strong behaviour pattern that is repeated over and over again. Habits may develop as entertainment for a bored child or, more commonly, as a coping mechanism to soothe anxiety. Sucking is a normal phenomenon during early infancy. Thumb-sucking when the child is hungry, disturbed and lonely, or is satisfying his urge for sucking, is a perfectly acceptable and normal phenomenon in children less than a year old.

What is the cause?

In infants, thumb-sucking is a common self-comforting behaviour that has pleasurable associations with feedings and cessation of hunger. The behaviour may linger into childhood because of these positive associations.

A hungry child may not only put his thumb, but his whole hand into his mouth. Sometimes the child is able to finish his bottle very quickly and since he has nothing else to do, he sucks his thumb. This is because sucking is soothing and comforting.

Usually babies who are breastfed are less likely to suck their thumbs than those who are bottle-fed. This is because a baby gets his milk more quickly through a bottle and is not able to fully satisfy the sucking urge. So he resorts to thumb-sucking. A breastfed baby may also suck his thumb if his sucking instinct is not fully satisfied. Children who do not suck their thumb before the age of one, seldom do it later.

An older child is often unaware that he is sucking the thumb. A child is not likely to spend time sucking his thumb if he finds his home life occupying and interesting. It is often an emotional problem that makes him suck his thumb. If the child is content, well fed and has playthings to occupy himself with, he will soon stop sucking his thumb.

What if the child continues to suck her thumb?

It is perfectly normal for a young child to suck her thumb or bite her nails. Sucking the thumb for a little while when falling asleep or when the child is tired should be allowed. Most schoolchildren have these habits. These unconscious, nervous habits are usually caused by tension. Do not try to stop your child through force or ridicule. The child will learn self-control by herself, as she grows older. She will become more conscious of her appearance and learn socially appropriate behaviour.

- Calmly point out what you do not like about the behaviour and why. This approach can be used with children as young as 3. Do not scold or lecture her. Punishment, ridicule or criticism could cause the behaviour to worsen.

- Involve the child in the process of breaking the habit. Ask your child what she thinks she could do to stop the habit or whether she wants to stop the habit.

- Children have a lot of energy. Give them paper, pencil, clay or mud for modelling, building blocks and other things to do. This will keep them occupied. If, after the age of five, a child sucks his thumb frequently without any obvious reason, consult your doctor for a check-up and then perhaps take the child to a child psychologist.

Help your child quit the habit

As children grow and develop, their need to suck usually goes away, most often by the time they are 6 to 8 years old. Severe emotional upsets or stress-related problems might cause the child to suck her thumb or use a pacifier for a long time. It is also possible that the child may be one of the very few who cannot seem to stop. However, most children stop daytime sucking habits when they begin school due to peer pressure. The same children might still use sucking as a way of going to sleep or calming themselves when they are upset. This is usually done in private and causes no harm either emotionally or physically. Putting too much pressure on the child to stop can cause more harm than good.

To help a child quit thumb-sucking, the first step is to ignore them! Most often, it will disappear with time. Harsh words, teasing or punishment may upset the child, and the habit will get worse. Punishment is not an effective way to get rid of habits. Older children (more than 3 years of age) may use sucking to relieve boredom. Try getting the child involved with an activity that she finds interesting. Rewarding good behaviour is the best way to bring about change. Praise and reward the child when she does not suck her thumb or use the pacifier.

If the above measures do not work, a paediatrician might recommend trying a reminder such as covering the thumb with a plastic strip or 'thumb guard' which is an adjustable plastic cap taped to the thumb. The child should be directly involved with the treatment chosen. Before using these methods, be sure to explain them to the child. If they make the child afraid or tense, stop them at once.

Does thumb-sucking affect the teeth?

A vigorous thumb-sucker can harm her teeth – the upper teeth will protrude forward while the lower tend to be drawn inwards or backwards. Since this habit is mainly in children under 5 years of age and the harm is done primarily to the milk teeth, one need not worry too much about it. However, if this habit persists beyond the age of five, the permanent teeth will also be affected, leading to expensive dental treatment for malformed teeth.

When to seek professional help?

Most habits are self-limiting and do not require professional help. But if the habit affects your child's physical or social functioning or persists even after you have tried all possible techniques, the behaviour may have a more serious emotional or physical cause. In these situations, you should consult your paediatrician or a mental health professional.

Toys for young children

Play and children

Children learn from the time they are born and parents or guardians are primarily responsible for providing quality experiences from which their children learn. Play is essential for learning in children. Parents often want to know about appropriate toys, books and computer or video games because they know that these tools may be important for their child's development.

Toys bring parents and children together in play. Early brain development is enhanced through these relationships. It is important for parents to understand the role of play in all areas of development, including cognitive, language, social, physical and emotional development. Toys should never be used as a substitute for love and unconditional attention from parents and other caregivers; toys enhance these interactions. When adults participate in the play of children, learning is enhanced. A child's self-esteem and level of mastery are also enhanced when adults participate in play. Parents are able to observe the skills in their child and also help in expanding them.

All children benefit from toys that promote safe physical activity. But some toys pose emotional or social risks. Graphic depictions of violence presented in an interactive way, such as in some computer or video games, can lead to acts of violence by the child. Although video games are rated, even those deemed for 'everyone' may contain significant violence. Toy weapons or other toys that promote violence should be discouraged. Parents should also consider whether a toy promotes any negative racial, cultural or gender stereotypes. The toys parents provide (or do not provide) send children a message about what is valued.

People marketing toys claim that specific toys will facilitate specific developmental milestones. There is no scientific evidence to suggest that a particular toy is necessary or sufficient for optimal learning. These advertisements can promote misinformation, inappropriate expectations and unnecessary expenditure. It could lead to parents feeling guilty when they cannot afford or they choose not to make such purchases. Just because a product is in the market does not mean it is safe. The characteristics of the toy, how the toy might be used or abused and the amount of supervision or help needed will determine its safety level or appropriate needs for use. It is important for parents to be familiar about toy safety guidelines.

Guidelines for parents and caregivers

- Most educational toys are those that encourage the interaction of an adult with a child in supportive, unconditional play. Toys should never be considered as substitutes for the attention of parents.
- Children should be provided with safe, affordable toys that are developmentally appropriate. Include toys that help to promote learning and growth in all areas of development and encourage creativity.
- Those toys should be avoided that discourage children from using their imagination. Social, emotional and cognitive skills are developed and enhanced when children use play to work out real-life problems.
- Use books and magazines to play and read together.
- Be skeptical of educational or developmental claims made by advertisers, especially claims of intellectual enhancement through certain toys.
- There are some toys that promote violence or negative social, racial or gender stereotypes. These toys are not recommended for children.
- It is good to limit video and computer games. The total screen time, including television and computer use, should be less than 1 to 2 hours per day. Children younger than 5 years should play with computer or video games only if they are developmentally appropriate, and a parent or caregiver should accompany the child.
- Toys should be made of safe nontoxic material. They should not have sharp edges. Small toys or toys which can easily be dismantled into parts should not be given to infants or toddlers as they may put them in their mouth. Toys should be stored safely.

Behaviour

1. Why doesn't my son respond when we talk to him?

Q. My son is 7 months old. He is aware of sounds, but when we call him or talk to him, he responds only sometimes while ignoring us most of the times. He keeps looking at different things or elsewhere. It seems that he is not able to understand that we are speaking to him. Is this behaviour normal or do I need to be concerned?

A. Babies communicate in many ways. They would look at you of course, but will also snuggle up to you and make gurgling sounds to express contentment and so on. Is your child doing this?

Does he turn to locate a sound? Does he appear to hear the music that is played or sung for him? If you are in doubt, you could get his hearing checked. Remedial work, if it is necessary, is better if started early. However, there may be no hearing problem. Infants are interested in looking at bright coloured objects and things that make a noise or move. Normally, the face of the mother or other caregivers is the most interesting thing for the child.

Different children will have different pace of development, which would fall into the category of normal. However, if you continue to have doubts, do consult a kind doctor or psychologist, who can guide you. Some babies may be so engrossed in what they are doing or watching that they may really ignore your voice despite hearing it.

2. How can I control my unruly daughter?

Q. My 20-month-old daughter is very active. She is a rebel but unusually smart. She understands perfectly what we ask her to do, but she refuses to

finish any task. She is very restless and does not have enough patience even when playing. She ignores all toys and uses everything that she knows is forbidden to her. Is this kind of behaviour normal? Is my daughter likely to become a toddler with hyperkinetic disorder?

A. Children are often smarter than we think! It seems your daughter is trying to test as to how far she can go. You should be firm and define limits. Be consistent in what you say 'no' to. The child will learn desirable actions if you are firm and consistent. Try to serve as good role models by observing patience and calmness yourself. It is premature to say if your child will turn out to be hyperactive, as most 2-year-olds have a lot of energy and curiosity, which can be a challenge to the parents. But your handling and disciplining efforts will surely help avoid negative trends.

3. How can I enhance my child's communication skills?

Q. I am poor in the use of Hindi language since I am from Southern India. I got married to a Hindi-speaking person but have yet not picked up the language. I am afraid about my daughter who is 16 months old. How can I teach her the language? She wants to interact with other kids and convey messages through me but I can't say anything. Even small kids here speak fluently. My husband is generally out. I am in a dilemma. Please help, I feel very lonely. What all should I do to develop my child's communication skills?

A. As your daughter grows up and starts moving around, she will pick up the language that others are speaking. As you may know, children learn the language they hear. You should also talk in your own language to her, tell her stories and sing songs. The mother tongue is learnt without an effort.

Children will learn Hindi or any other language used, as they play with other children. Anyway, at 16 months, most children use only a few words, although they understand a lot more. So your child is not at a disadvantage yet.

You could also start learning spoken Hindi yourself from a Hindi-speaking woman in the area, perhaps from a retired schoolteacher. You will find that Hindi is a very easy language to learn. You can also borrow class I Hindi books and teach yourself. When your Hindi-speaking neighbours find that you are keen to learn their language, at least one or two of them will be willing to help. When your child is with others, she will learn to communicate. There is no cause for worry. In fact your child will be able to help you to speak Hindi, in a year from now.

4. I feel guilty leaving my infant with my in-laws, what should I do?

Q. I had to leave my child at home with my in-laws when she was 10 weeks old. I tried coming home to spend time with her as much as possible. My sister-in-law, older than me, does not have a child and lives some distance away from us. She used to come and play with my child at least twice a week. Now whenever my sister-in-law comes home my child refuses to come to me except when she is hungry. She is 7 months old now and my in-laws want me to stop feeding as I am weak. But I feel very insecure. Also, I feel guilty about letting my baby in other people's care. What should I do?

A. It is quite normal for you to want to be the most important person in your baby's life. It is also quite normal for the baby to want to stay with those who play with her and make her feel good. Your situation (working outside the home) makes it necessary for other family members to spend time with your baby. Do not resent it; rather be happy that the child has the possibility of good care, even in your absence. However, if you wish to have more time for your child, see if you can take up a part-time job or reduce some responsibilities at work in order to spend more time at home. If that is not possible, let your mother-in-law and sister-in-law give the baby the attention and care that she needs. As she grows up, the child will be attached to you as well. Most children in our country thrive under multiple mothering or having motherly care from more than one person. Relax and enjoy when your child is with you.
(*See also* page 24)

5. How can we help our child to adjust in a different culture?

Q. I am an Indian and have taken up a full-time employment in Oman 3 months ago. I have shifted from Delhi along with my wife and a 2-year-old son. The problem relates to my son's personal development. People in Oman are local Omanis or South Indians, Bangladeshis, Pakistanis, Filipinos or Sri Lankans. There is practically no culture of people mixing around with each other. I am aware that my 2-year-old son should now mix with other children of his age group, which will benefit him in his personal and mental development. But there are no children of his age group here, nor is there any mingling of families due to which he has been within the boundaries of our house, with only my wife and me for company. We take him out to the

park, markets or for a walk in the evening occasionally and he seems to enjoy the time outdoors. Is this the right age for him to go to a kindergarten school so that he is able to mix with children? Or should we wait for him to grow up to the age of 3? What kind of routine should we maintain so that the environmental deficiencies do not hamper my child's personality?

A. I am glad to come upon parents who take a keen interest in their child's development. However, I find it very surprising that you find no culture of people mixing around in Muscat. Maybe you need to find ways of enlarging your social circle gradually. The very fact that you, as an Indian, have bracketed South Indians along with people of other countries perhaps reflects your Delhi-centric approach. Travel normally gives us opportunities to meet people different from ourselves and to appreciate their customs. But it takes time and you have had only 3 months. A good way to start is by making friends with neighbours and with colleagues in the office/factory. The families could meet on weekends. That will enlarge your son's world. But all these attempts will be successful only if you have respect for people of different cultures.

Most KGs and nursery schools will admit children who are over 3 years of age. You could find out if there is a playgroup for 2-year-olds, operating from someone's house. But the child will be comfortable away from the mother only for a period of an hour or so.

There are several play activities that you can organize at home. These include music, moving to rhythm, colouring with chalk or crayon, etc. Let the child's interest and pace decide what you give him. Do not try to make him learn up facts or be older than his age. Children love to hear stories and read picture books. Give the child a chance to run around the house and in the park. Get him a soft ball to push around.

A child's development is best attained through playing with the right kind of play materials and having warm and supportive adults looking after him. The child likes to be talked to and treated as a person. There is no specific formula except parental love and thoughtful caring.

6. How should I control my child's indefinite crying?

Q. My son is 15 months old. He has become so stubborn that if we stop him for anything he starts crying. He keeps crying until we take him in our arms. Due to this, we are forced not to scold, beat or give any harsh punishment. How should I control him?

A. Being a parent is a responsibility, but it is also a joy equal to no other.

It appears to me that you are feeling the weight of being a parent, without the delight that goes with having a child. Children do learn to make things happen. If they do not get parental attention, they may cry till somebody appears and picks them up. Their crying is also a message: the child could be too hot, or too cold, hungry or wet, with colic or some other discomfort. These messages from the baby should not be treated as 'stubbornness' (it is such a negative sounding word), but as the child's intelligent attempt to get your attention.

I am a little surprised that you say you are forced not to scold, beat or give any punishment. Why would you want to scold the child? He has probably not yet developed enough language to understand your scolding anyway. Hitting a 15-month-old? I can't believe that you feel unhappy because you cannot hit him. Please restrain yourselves and find out why you are getting angry with the child. I would need to know more facts before giving you definite advice. But I make some general suggestions. Perhaps both parents work and the child wants to be held and cuddled when they are available to him. This is natural and very good for the ties of affection between the child and the parents. I think there is no point in treating him like a cadet in the army. He is just a baby, an infant, who wants assurance that he is loved by his parents. Sometimes children may be weak or underweight and therefore cry all the time. If that is the case, you should worry about his nutrition, not his discipline. Just check with your doctor that the child is in fine health. Why would you want to give him harsh punishment? Every message can be conveyed gently and with affection, playfully and with concern.

Try and spend more time with your child. Talk to him, sing to him, dance with him and tell him stories. You will find that he is no longer unhappy. Get suitable picture books and toys for the child. Treat your parenting with more energy and joy and the problems will disappear. Children will discipline themselves and you do not need to be a policeman to them.

7. How can I prevent my child from sucking her lower lip?

Q. My daughter is 3 years old. She has a habit of sucking her lower lip since she was a year old. She continuously sucks her lip and also rubs her fingers on my mouth. She does this before going to sleep and at other times, like while watching a movie. She is a clever child and can understand everything except this. This act of hers is very irritating and sometimes I beat her for this, as she even touches lips of others, apart from me, who are friendly to her.

A. A habit can sometimes become a source of security for the child. Instead of beating her for it or trying reasoning, simply try to ignore her or distract her when she shows undesirable behaviour. And when she does not show undesirable behaviour, give her love and attention.

You can even predict when she may touch your lips; try to change your posture to be away from her. Try to gradually mould her behaviour away from firstly touching others' lips, and then her own. An old-fashioned home remedy for this kind of behaviour would be to put the paste of fresh neem leaves on her lip. It is bitter, non-toxic and can do no harm.

8. Does my child too have attention deficit disorder?

Q. **My son will be 3 years old next year. His teacher at the daycare is concerned with his lack of ability to stay on a task. He frequently interrupts his dad and me when we are reading books to him, but only to try and read them himself. He is stubborn and does not like to eat much. He is extremely active and sits still only to watch movies. What can we do to increase his ability to stay on a task and focus? Our 8-year-old daughter is a slow learner and has ADHD [attention-deficient hyperactivity disorder] but my son has none of the symptoms she had, except for defiance and inability to stay on a task.**

A. How much concentration and focus do you expect from a 2-year-old? From your account, he watches movies, tries to read from the book that you are reading out to him and is very active. It sounds like he is a healthy, bright child. If you read any textbook on child development, you will find that 2-year-olds do move rapidly from one task to another.

But since a professional psychologist has assessed your daughter for ADHD, it would be desirable to get your son assessed too. Each child is different from another and not all problems are genetic. Though one hopes that your son does not suffer from any disorder, it would still require professional assessment to come to a proper conclusion. After the assessment, kindly follow the advice given by the psychologist. The staff at the daycare is probably using the same methods for infants that they have learned for use with 4- and 5-year-olds. It may be good to give your son a lot of opportunity for running around and other vigorous physical activity.

9. Why is my child more attached to my mother-in-law?

Q. **I am a working woman and have a 2-year-old son. I feel that my son is**

very attached to my mother-in-law who takes care of him when I go to work. The problem is that she never allows him to play with small children. I would like to know whether this will affect him in future and I would also like to know how I could make him feel happy so that he also likes to stay with me? My mother-in-law does not have an understanding nature and she always tries to keep him away from me.

A. You leave the child with your mother-in-law because you need her help while you are away at work. It is obvious that the child will be attached to her. Your mother-in-law may not be finding it easy to allow him to interact with other children. The point is that if you take the decision to leave the child with her, you will have to accept the fact that the child may be more attached to her. You will also have to accept that she is doing you a favour. She is obviously older and has her own experience and wisdom. You may suggest any changes in her parenting style with affection and respect, but you cannot demand her to change. If you are so suspicious of her intentions and impact, maybe you can explore the possibility of leaving the child at a creche or daycare centre. Other factors that affect the upbringing of the child are the role of the father, you as a mother and the total family environment. (*See also* page 21)

10. Why does my daughter hold her urine till she wets herself?

Q. My 3-year-old daughter is very stubborn. Whenever she has to go to the toilet, she holds herself and that is when we realize that she needs to go. But when we offer to accompany her, she keeps running from one room to another hiding, but does not go to the toilet, till she wets herself. I am not sure whether it is that she cannot control herself and is afraid to admit, or she is just being stubborn. She was fine a year ago till my mother was taking care of her. But she got busy with my ill father, so my daughter was left without her care. After that we have put her on Pampers. What kind of food will refresh her appetite? What is the solution for her wetting problem?

A. Your daughter seems to have had some experience that has upset her. Normally children who have been toilet trained do not go back to wetting themselves during the daytime. Please do take her to see a psychologist or psychiatrist, who will be able to help her. Please do not scold or punish her. Maybe she had a very unpleasant experience when she went to the toilet. It would need patience and skill to find out what the problem has been. If you could spend the next couple of months with her, during the main part of the day and night, it might reassure her. But since you have not given details, I am not able to label the problem or to suggest measures you can take. If you are kind and gentle, she will pick up confidence in herself. Play with her and cook special dishes for her, which are non-spicy and look interesting. Food cooked without too many spices and served attractively in small portions will be good for your child. You must realize that her lack of interest in eating is related to everything else that is happening to her. Spend at least an hour before her bedtime telling her stories, playing some music or reading to her.

11. How should I take care of my daughter after my divorce?

Q. I am 30 years old and got divorced 6 months ago. My daughter is 18 months old. My wife refused to accept our daughter and I took custody of her. Since I am working, I am not able to devote much time to her. My parents who are living in another city look after her. How should I bring up the child and make a bright career for her?

A. I am glad that you have your parents to take care of your young daughter. Make sure she is happy. See her as often as you can so that she forms a bond with you. At this stage, she just needs good nutrition and care, play activities and affection. These will be the foundation for her life. It seems too early to worry about her career. She could be sent to a nursery school near the home after she is 3 years old.

12. How can we make our son brave?

Q. My son is 1-and-a-half years old. He is active and playful, but is scared of children elder to him, especially when they shout and laugh loudly. He avoids going to them. He doesn't resist if something is snatched from him and turns towards me for help. We have tried to explain to him about how to develop resistance and courage. We have also explained that he should not get frightened and be brave. We have observed that our neighbour's children come over to play with my son's toys, but my son keeps distance and in spite of our telling him to play with them, he keeps watching them with a sense of fear. We know that he is too young to understand what we say, but how can we make him brave? In the long run, if he continues with this attitude, we fear that he will be exploited. How can we help him to defend his belongings and cultivate braveness?

A. Perhaps you worry too much about the long run. Let your child grow up and decide when he wants to protect his toys from others. Each child is born with a temperament and a way of doing things. Sometimes children change totally after a certain age or experience. But it is better to let them work it out. If your son comes to you for help, you should of course give it. Perhaps he had some fearful experience when he was an infant. He will gradually get used to loud noises and boisterous friends. At the age of 18 months, children generally like to play with adults (who will be sensitive to their needs) or with children who are much older and at an age when they can look after the younger ones. It is only when they are 3-plus that children play with their age mates and, even then, under supervision of adults. Give him lots of opportunities to play rough and tumble games with you. As he grows bigger and stronger, he will be comfortable with other children.

13. Why does my son behave violently with other children?

Q. My son is 2-and-a-half years old. At times, he behaves very differently. Once he went to play football, but when other children came to play with him, he purposely threw the ball in the bushes, so that no one could take the ball. This has happened 3–4 times. Also, when we have guests at home, he tries to harm their children, by biting them, stamping their feet, throwing sand on their head or just hitting with a toy on the head. I am very worried about his violent outbursts. Please advise.

A. Your child does seem to have a problem about sharing his toys or space with others. Some of it is age-related. Children become more sociable after they complete 3. He will improve in a few months. Nevertheless, he seems to have very physical ways of expressing himself. You will have to spend more time with him, talking to him and encouraging him to express himself in words. He should be rewarded with praise and hugs when he behaves well. If the problems continue, you could try and see a psychologist, to assure yourself that his behaviour is within acceptable limits. Teach him that all games are more enjoyable when played with other children. (*See also* page 100)

14. Why does my son keep screaming and crying all the time?

Q. My 2-year-old son is the youngest of the three children I have. He has

always been demanding. But ever since he turned 2 he has become worse. He screams and cries all through the day. If he wants juice, he will scream for it over and over, and become louder as he gets close to me. If I am on the phone or working on the computer, he will grab my face and make me look at him. But if I tell him to hold on, he screams even louder. Every door has to be closed at all times otherwise he keeps screaming 'door, door' until it's shut. Sometimes I think he has obsessive–compulsive disorder (OCD). He is horrified of bugs. The other day I had to put him in the front seat of the car because he kept crying 'bug' while seated in the back seat. But there wasn't any bug around. He refuses to sleep in his room, and if I put him in his bed, he vomits. Please advise. He is the sweetest of all three of my children. He's loving and affectionate, but he's driving me crazy.

A. It is better to try and find out why your child gets upset than to treat it as a behavioural problem. For this, you may need to see a doctor, psychologist or counsellor. It seems to me that the child has had some experience, which has scared him (even a horrible TV programme could have done it) or that he has become sensitive to certain things. I cannot put a label on it with the amount of information you have given. He obviously has a low tolerance for frustration. So instead of letting him scream, it might be better to attend to his needs, till he gets better.

If he is affectionate and sweet as you say, find out what has happened to make him so demanding. Deal with all issues gently, not as if the child is in a court of law. Do consult a suitable expert.

15. Why does my child not share with others?

Q. My son is going to turn 3 in two months. His problem is that he always cries. Whatever he wants he expresses it in tears. He won't give his things to his own cousins. Both of us are quite irritated about this. I am sometimes harsh with him. Please tell me how to tackle this situation?

A. You seem to expect too much from a child who is not even 3 yet. Your son is too young to understand the concept of sharing. Getting irritated with him would not be of any help. The best option is to explain to him the benefits of sharing through stories, and praise him whenever he makes an effort to share. Be gentle in your handling of the child and as he grows older, he will develop the confidence to share his toys and books.

Fussy eaters

16. How can I make my daughter eat everything?

Q. My daughter is 3 years old. She is 86 cm tall and weighs 10 kg. She is very active and intelligent, but she is a fussy eater and she doesn't eat by herself. This combination leads to my shouting and cursing her. She hates milk, cereals, fruits, etc. We have to force, shout, or tell her stories to make her eat. Each meal takes about half an hour to 2 hours. If left to her, she will neither drink milk nor eat more than 2–3 bites. She likes chips, ladyfinger, namak pare, etc. I generally avoid chips unless we are out of home. I give her ladyfinger 2–3 times in a week and namak paare once a day, as snacks. I prepare nutritious and a variety of things like poha, upma, parantha, all seasonal vegetables and fruits. We eat everything and make her eat with us. She likes curd a lot. But she gets throat infection, so I can't give her that. She does not relish paneer. She used to drink milk from the bottle from 1 year to 2-and-a-half years of age, but it's a struggle from the glass. I dread waking her up in the morning and getting her ready for school. Milk takes an hour and she does not take any solids. Her father was like her in his childhood. Is the behaviour hereditary? How can I make her eat by herself? My husband is against taking help of any professional in this respect. All this is affecting my behaviour. At times I don't feel like talking to my daughter or loving her. Please help.

A. Since your child has some food preferences, there is no harm in including them in her diet everyday. If she likes chips, make that a part of the meal, at least once a day, so that some calories go in. If she hates milk and likes curd, give her curd. It is not scientifically established that curd gives one a cold. Only, you should make sure that the curd is not sour or too cold. Serve her curd at or just a little below room temperature.

While some children eat by themselves even at 18 months, other children take their time. There is no harm in feeding your child, but without shouting at her or forcing her. Make mealtimes a little playful, with stories and conversations.

Introduce new foods gradually and let her taste them and decide if she likes something. Maybe she would drink milk if you added some cocoa powder to it. Sometimes children eat a dosa or chapatti if it is made into funny shapes, like a cat or a flower! Instead of putting all your energy into getting your child to eat by herself, do something by which she has the required nutrients. Gradually she will put on weight and start eating on her own.

In the mornings, let her go to school on a full stomach rather than a half full stomach. I am convinced that you provide a variety of foods on the table, but most children under the age of 8 do not seem to relish upma or poha. They prefer something crisp, which they can pick up and eat. It seems to me to be simply a matter of adjusting your expectations for a few months. You are interested in her being healthy and happy. To ensure this, you cannot enact a semi-tragedy every morning. Relax! Children do grow up!

17. Is it acceptable for my child to ask for snacks from neighbours?

Q. My son is 2 years and 3 months old. My wife being a housewife stays with him all day. During the day, he runs to the neighbour's house and prefers to play there. He also eats snacks before and after lunch at their house. He asks for snacks from them. We find this very disturbing. Is this an acceptable behaviour for a 2-year-old? Do we need to control it, if yes, how should we go about it?

A. A 2-year-old child is too young to understand that it is not desirable to be as free at a neighbour's house as at home, especially if the neighbour is affectionate. Children want to spend time where they get love and attention. Setting a routine for him for his meals and playtime is important. Explaining in simple and direct terms that too much food at the neighbour's house is not desirable could help. By observation, you would know whether he enjoys their food especially, or the chance to eat it with children of his age. In any case, you should stop worrying about it if your neighbours are comfortable with it.

18. Why has my daughter stopped eating in my absence?

Q. My daughter is 1-and-a-half years old. She is staying at my in-law's house with her mother for the past 3 months. I go and visit them regularly over the weekends. But since the past one week, she is not playing actively and she refuses to eat. Her body temperature is normal and she has developed cough. The doctor has diagnosed upper respiratory infection (URI). How can we increase her appetite? What is the reason for her inactivity? Is it due to my absence? She keeps on murmuring daddy, daddy during my absence.

A. Your daughter seems to be suffering from a health problem, for which appropriate treatment must be sought. It is also possible that she is feeling insecure due to being away from home and you. Since there must be valid reasons for your wife and child staying away from you, you must ensure that they do not feel neglected. Make sure that your child is happily engaged in supervised play during the day. Food that is softly cooked and not over-spiced should be given to her 4–6 times a day. Processed foods and cola drinks should not be given. If her problem persists, consult a children's doctor. Lack of appetite could be temporary, because of the cough.

School issues

19. Why does my daughter remain silent in school?

Q. My daughter is 2 years and 10 months old. She studies in baby nursery. She is going to the school for the past 4–5 months. Initially, she was very cranky at school, but now she doesn't cry while going to school. Her teacher and the van driver told me that she doesn't speak at all in school. She is doing this for the past 2 months. I was admitted to the hospital for a week for a hernia surgery. Initially, I thought it was because of this. But it has been almost 2 months that she is like this in school. At home she is perfectly fine, she talks, sings and dances. But when I ask her anything about school, she doesn't have much to tell. The teachers in her school are quite friendly. How should I handle this situation?

A. Though social norms in our country make it common to send a 2-year-old to school, it can prove to be a traumatic experience for the child. Since the child is still in the process of establishing a secure attachment with the mother figure, it can result in separation anxiety and insecurity. In the case of your daughter, it seems that she is not enjoying the school atmosphere. Absence of crying does not mean that she has adjusted. Besides, there is your own illness and hospitalization.

You should try to talk to her and understand her feelings. Try to assess if there is something that is making her afraid at school, whether there is something about other children or any teacher that upsets her. Change of school can be considered if you find any concrete reason.

On your part, you should try and make her feel secure that you love and accept her as she is, and that you are in good health now. Spend more quality time with her. Some children are talkative at home but quiet at school. If she is happy and active, maybe there is nothing to worry. The best policy is to wait and watch. If things do not improve, you can consult a child psychologist for psychological evaluation and help.

20. Will leaving the child in a creche hamper his mental growth?

Q. We are working parents. We have a 7-and-a-half-month-old baby boy. Currently we keep him at a creche for 5 days a week. The lady who runs the creche is MSc in child psychology. Our baby is very active and always busy doing something. But, when we take him to the creche or bring him back from there he becomes sad and unhappy. Will it affect his psychology in the long-term? I have a better job than my wife. Should my wife quit the job? How should we handle the issue?

A. I think you are lucky to have a creche (daycare centre for infants and young children) available, which is operated by a qualified person. Why don't you talk to the person in charge to see how your baby is adjusting? If he is quite happy most of the time, he has already adjusted. Maybe, with the permission of the people managing the creche, you could spend a couple of hours in the adjoining room, without being seen by your son, to reassure yourselves that all is well. Some creches do not permit this because the babies may get upset seeing some parent-like adults and start missing their own.

Without knowing all the circumstances, I will not be able to advise the child's mother whether to give up her job or not. There will be no damage to the child's physical or mental health if the creche in which the child spends 5 days a week is clean, well run and baby-friendly. You have the whole weekend to spend with your little son. When you are with the child, give him a lot of cuddling and holding. Play with him, talk to him, feed him and bathe him – all this, cheerfully and with love. The baby should feel secure and be certain of your love. If he does, he can face being separated from you for short periods and will know that you will come back. His showing sadness is natural, but once you leave him and go away, he will get adjusted to your absence. It is thus important to satisfy yourselves about the suitability of the creche and to find out from the caregivers about your child's adjustment to the creche. In the long-term, the unqualified love that you give him is the most important input in his life. Separation experiences will always be there, but can be handled when relationships are good.

21. Is it all right to put an 11-month-old in a toddlers' club?

Q. My son is almost 11 months old. I am thinking of putting him in a toddlers club run by a playschool wherein the child has to attend the sessions thrice a week for one hour each day. The mother has to accompany the child for all the sessions. The school basically has three different rooms. One is a language room, where there will be story-telling, teaching different colours, etc. The second one is the drama room, where they hold puppet shows, have a doll house, etc. And the third is the motor room, where they encourage the children to coordinate muscle movements of different body parts. Will these kind of activities and interaction with children of his age group help him for his future growth? Is he too small for such activities?

A. From your description of the toddlers' club, it does seem as if they would pitch the activities to the age level of the children and that it could be a lot of fun. It would be an opportunity for the child to be in the same room with others of his age and for the mother to meet other young mothers. It will also be a chance to find out how professionals handle the issues related to the education and amusement of young children. Also, it is only three times a week and with the mother present.

A good home can of course provide many of these activities, if the mother is talented and has time. This is often not the case. I know of many parents who leave the TV and a caregiver, or even a grandmother who watches TV all day, to take care of the child.

You will have to consider the alternatives and make a decision. If the activities in the playschool are planned for his age group, he is sure to benefit from them. It is not only the future that you have to worry about, it is the present. Consult your family and friends and make the best decision in the interests of the child and his situation.

22. How can I spare more time to teach my daughter?

Q. My daughter is 2 years and 10 months old. I am a working mother and have a busy working schedule. I meet her in the evenings and spend quality time with her. In between I talk to her on phone for nearly 2 hours everyday. She stays with my mother where a lot of people are there to take care of her. She gets a lot of attention when she is there. She is joining school this year. I know that this is the time to give foundation to her future but, due to my busy schedule, I can't give her more attention. Please suggest some alternative

ways and how do I spend this limited time with her, which will be useful for her for learning?

A. Your child seems to be spending most of the day in the warm company of the grandparents and other relatives. That is an excellent substitute for the care you would be giving. It is a little surprising to me that you spend 2 hours on the phone talking to her. If you can spare that much time, perhaps you could also commit to fewer hours on the job and have more time for face-to-face interaction with your daughter.

She is not even 3 years old yet. There is no need to teach her. Children like to learn things through playing with toys, chalks and crayons, household objects like spoons and cups and of course playing with children and adults. Speech is learnt through listening and talking, concepts through trying out things and observing. Opportunities for all these activities, including some music to hear and some music to sing, activities for movement, picture books, puppets, rag-dolls, etc. can be provided.

The child needs to develop trust in you and other caregivers. She needs affection, nutritious low-spiced home-cooked food and plenty of sleep. That is the best investment you can make. Teaching the child to recite or perform before others does not necessarily provide the foundation. In fact, it can do just the opposite, forcing the child to merely perform for adult approval.

The best building blocks are the intangibles of parental love, age-appropriate activities for the child and the presence of adults who care and allow the child to grow naturally and with self-confidence. There is no other secret formula!

23. Do daycare centres impact a child's development?

Q. My son is 2 years and 9 months old. Since I am working and I don't have anybody to take care of him, I have to leave him in a childcare centre. I have been doing this since he was 9 months old. Will there be any drawback in such a child who is brought up in a childcare centre? My son has a habit of thumb-sucking since he was 2 months old. I breastfed him till he was 6 months old but later he totally refused to take mother's milk. This forced me to give a substitute after two continuous days of efforts to feed him my milk. When I consulted my doctor he asked me to just leave him as it is and he will automatically leave this habit once he goes to school. How do I cut down his habit of thumb-sucking? He is also hyperactive and unable to concentrate.

He doesn't sit for even two minutes if we take him to a new place like friend's/relative's house. Either I or my husband have to run behind him to keep a watch on him.

A. The impact of daycare centre on a child's development depends on two aspects:

- quality of environment and care in the centre, and
- quality of interaction with parents.

If the daycare centre is caring and hygienic and you as parents are giving adequate time, love and attention to the child, there should be no need to worry.

Thumb-sucking becomes a source of concern when the child reaches the age of getting permanent teeth. It is better to gradually divert his attention when you find him sucking his thumb. But do not make him too conscious of it, as he would then do it behind your back.

A 2–3-year-old child is usually very active and parents may mistake normal activity levels for hyperactivity. It is best to let the problem be diagnosed by a child psychologist and then take remedial steps as advised. (*See also* pages 14, 19)

Sleep concerns

24. Can I make my child sleep separately?

Q. My baby boy will complete 7 months by the end of this month. For the past 15 days we have started to let him sleep in a separate bed (in the same bedroom though) whereas earlier he used to sleep with the mother. He is comfortable with sleep now as well. Is it okay to let the baby sleep separately from his mother so early?

A. Your decision seems quite good. If the baby is comfortable and sleeps well in his own cradle or crib, that is fine!

Though, I would suggest a few points to be kept in mind. Make sure that the baby is warm and that he does not kick off the coverings. If possible, a zipped-up warm sleeping suit is the best thing. But you should also make sure that the baby is not too hot, as that could also cause discomfort. Be willing to adjust the rules to his health. If he is sick or upset for any reason, he may want more cuddling and comforting.

In western countries, parents tend to put the baby to sleep in a totally separate room, if they have the space. (When I was a student in the US, I used to babysit for families in the neighbourhood and it was an amazement to see each child in a separate bedroom, in rich homes.) Every system works, with some plus and minus points. I think the arrangement you have made to let the child sleep in his cradle in the same room seems to be sound and it generally is more acceptable in Indian families. Your responding to the baby's needs for feeds or toiletting will be immediate and that ensures his comfort. Actually there are no rules, only the advice to make the best arrangement under given conditions. What works best for you is all right.

25. Why does my child take so long to go to sleep?

Q. **My daughter is 2 years and 3 months old. She has a problem going to sleep. In fact it takes too long for us to put her to sleep. She never sleeps on her own at night. She is hyperactive and has learned to speak very fast; she can speak her mother tongue very well and sing many nursery rhymes. She can tell colours and shapes but doesn't understand the concept of sharing and is little scared of kids of the same age but takes very good care of young children and plays well with grown-up kids. Can you tell me what can be the problem, if any?**

A. Your daughter seems to be a normal, healthy and intelligent child. She is able to get along with other children, and the fact that she is more cautious with kids of her age is a natural behaviour in some children.

Regarding her sleeping pattern, perhaps you can try out the following:

- Make sure that she does not take a long nap in the afternoon.
- As night progresses, make sure that there is a gradual slowing down of noise and activities in the household.
- Too much of TV viewing should be discouraged. Put a limit on the time that she spends in front of a TV.
- Try to soothe her and sing a lullaby or play some soft music at bedtime.

Perhaps you are trying to teach her everything too soon. Let her play with toys of her choice.

26. Why does my baby girl not sleep when outside?

Q. **My baby girl is 9 months old and has a habit of refusing to sleep when she is somewhere outside. Whenever she is sleepy, she will cry non-stop. We tried carrying her, patting her to sleep, but it is of no use. We also tried putting her in the pram and closing the cover, but still she refuses to sleep. She has been like this since she was born. She can only sleep when she lies down on a mattress, carrying her bolster and with her thumb holding on to our fingers. Is there anyway I can put her to sleep when we are out? I have seen many young infants who sleep soundly in the arms of their parents or in the pram.**

A. Some babies are quicker to form habits than others. Your child's association of going to sleep is of the time and place, which is routine. Your child's refusal to sleep when out of the house, in parents' arms or in the pram could be the result of habituation. She is probably used to sleeping in a quiet place with no outside sounds. You can only get her out of this habit with a lot of patience and gradual effort. Some introspection may help in understanding if she is getting enough time for bonding with the mother. At this stage of infancy, children go through a phase of attachment formation and it is necessary to form a trusting relationship with the mother, before the child can get over an unfamiliar bedtime routine.

27. If kids watch their parents have sex, will it adversely affect them?

Q. We are an Indian couple based in Mauritius. We have 1-year-old twins (a boy and a girl) and our house is a 6-bedroom bungalow. We usually put the kids to sleep in our room as they cry. Once they are put to sleep, my wife and I have sex and intercourse for almost 3–4 hours. Sometimes the kids wake up and we both are so involved in our fantasy that we forget that the kids are watching us. Will this lead to any bad implications?

A. The majority of Indian families in the lower and lower middle class have no privacy. You are fortunate to have a large house. If it is possible, you might try making the room next to yours a nursery for the two children. Be with them till they fall asleep. They will get used to having a room of their own. Keep a low light on all night. You should check occasionally during the night to make sure that all is well with the babies. However, you are the best judge of when to start the process.

As they grow up, children do find out the facts about sex. But it might be better for the parents to select a suitable age when they are given the information. No dire consequences can be predicted of their sharing your bedroom, but do not be surprised if they imitate the approximate actions when they start attending a preschool or playgroup.

Preschoolers (3 to 5 years)

- Markers – Preschoolers (3 to 5 years)
- Dealing with fears
- Temper tantrums
- Sex education
- Fussy eaters
- Speech disorders
- Stammering ... and how to overcome it

- Difficult children
- Habits
- School issues
- Fussy eaters
- Parenting
- Speech disorders
- Sex education
- Miscellaneous

Markers – Preschoolers (3 to 5 years)

The third year

Physical and motor-skill markers

- Gains about 2.25 kg and grows about 3 inches
- Will improve social skills and will enjoy playing with other children
- Will comprehend the meaning of words such as 'on', 'under' and 'behind'
- Will be able to formulate quite complex sentences
- Will be able to draw a circle
- Has improved balance
- Has improved vision
- May have daytime control over bowel and bladder functions (may have night-time control as well)
- Can briefly balance on one foot
- May walk up the stairs with alternating feet
- Can construct a block tower of more than 9 cubes
- Can easily place tiny objects in a small opening

Sensory and cognitive markers

- Has a vocabulary of several hundreds of words
- Composes sentences of 3–4 words
- Frequently asks questions
- Can dress self, only requiring assistance with laces, buttons
- Has longer attention span
- Feeds self without difficulty
- Acts out social encounters through play activities
- Has less separation anxiety for short periods of time

The fourth year

Physical and motor-skill markers

- Gains weight at the rate of about 6 grams per day
- Grows to a height that is double the length at birth
- Shows improved balance
- Hops on one foot without losing balance
- Throws a ball overhand with coordination
- Can cut out a picture using paper scissors

Sensory and cognitive markers

- Has a vocabulary of over 1500 words
- Easily composes sentences of 4–5 words
- Can use the past tense
- Asks a lot of questions
- May use words that are not fully understood

- Learns and sings simple songs
- Tries to be very independent
- May show increased aggressive behaviour
- Commonly has imaginary playmates
- Lacks moral concepts of right and wrong

The fifth year

Physical and motor-skills markers

- May erupt the first permanent teeth but the majority of children do not get their first permanent teeth until age 6.
- Develops increased coordination
- Skips, jumps, and skates with good balance
- Maintains balance while standing on one foot with eyes closed
- Ties own shoelaces
- Shows increased skill with simple tools

Sensory and cognitive markers

- Vocabulary increases to over 2100 words
- Composes sentences of 6–8 words, and with all parts of speech
- Questions more deeply, addressing meaning and purpose
- Behaves more responsibly
- Outgrows earlier childhood fears
- Accepts the validity of other points of view
- Demonstrates increased mathematical skill
- Strongly identifies with the parent of the same sex

Dealing with fears

What is the cause?

All children have fears of one kind or another. Fear is an emotion just as love, happiness, anger, hurt and sadness. Babies are unpredictable. In the early days of their lives they are quite fearless. They go boldly into the great unknown. As the child grows older, her imagination and curiosity also develops. She learns the potential dangers of certain actions and objects and the reasons for it. As she makes these connections, her awareness makes her cautious and sometimes frightened.

It has been observed that these fears develop more often in children for whom feeding and toilet training have been contentious issues, or in those who have over-protective parents or who have been regularly warned or cautioned against doing certain things. On the other hand, some children are just born sensitive. They will slowly grow out of them with your understanding and help.

Fear of the dark

Fear of the dark is one of the most common childhood fears. This fear is common in adults too. If your child is scared of the dark you can indulge her by leaving her bedroom door open or leaving a night light on. Keep her well occupied with games and other activities throughout the day so that she has no time to brood on her fears. In time, she will realize that there is nothing to fear.

Tangible fears

Sometimes children develop fears of tangible objects such as dogs, cockroaches, water and men in uniform. It is not necessary for the child to have had a frightening experience with any of the objects of their fears. It will certainly not help them to overcome their fear by forcing them to confront the object of their fears. Children generally outgrow these fears themselves.

Fear of death

Some children are scared of death and dying. They cannot understand what happens to their pets or people who die. It is necessary for the parents to explain to the child that the deceased has gone up to God in heaven. On the other hand, parents can deal with death by saying that the person was old, weak and too tired to go on living. It is important that parents reassure their child that they will be around for years to come.

Fear at the movies

Some children begin to wail in the theatres and demand to be taken home.

Parents must remember that children below the age of 7 often find it difficult to separate fiction and reality because of their overactive imagination. Thus, movies may not be a good idea for children in this age group.

Fear of separation

Although separation anxieties are normal among infants and toddlers, they are not appropriate for older children or adolescents. They may represent symptoms of separation anxiety disorder. Children with separation anxiety may cling to their parent and have difficulty falling asleep by themselves at night. Their need to stay close to their parent or home may make it difficult for them to attend school or stay at friends' houses, or be in a room by themselves. Fear of separation can even lead to dizziness, nausea or palpitations.

Separation anxiety is often associated with symptoms of depression, such as sadness, withdrawal, apathy or difficulty in concentrating, and such children often fear that they or a family member might die. Young children experience nightmares or fears at bedtime.

Social phobias

Children with social phobias (also called social anxiety disorder) have a persistent fear of being embarrassed. They get embarrassed in social situations such as during a performance, or if they have to speak in class or in public, or get into conversation with others or eat, drink or write in public. Feelings of anxiety in these situations may produce physical reactions such as palpitations, tremors, sweating, diarrhoea, blushing, muscle tension, etc. Children may be afraid that others will notice their anxiety and consider them odd and make fun of them.

Divorce

At some point all children are afraid of being abandoned, but when parents separate, the fear of being left alone becomes all too real. The child may assume that since one parent has left, the other will too. Suddenly a child's natural desire to explore the world gets replaced by the anxiety of being left alone at home. Children of parents intending to divorce need extra care and they should be made to feel safe as the world can seem a threatening place to youngsters in such a situation. It is very important to handle the situation with sensitivity.

How to help the child?

While you may not understand the child's fear, it is very real to her. Ridiculing the fear or chastising your child for being a coward is not going to make the situation better. Encourage her to talk about her fears. You must instil confidence in her by assuring her that nothing bad is going to happen and that you are right there by her side. While it is important to be sympathetic, do not overdo it. Your child may get the message that her fears are justified. You can help the child develop the skills and confidence to overcome her fears.

The following steps will guide you in helping your child deal with her fears and anxieties.

- Recognize that the fear is real even if it seems trivial to you. It feels real to the child and it is causing her to feel anxious and afraid. Being able to talk about fears can help.
- Never belittle the fear as a way of forcing the child to overcome it. It will not make the fear go away. Let her know that both of you are there for her – whatever your differences as a couple.
- Parents who display frequent fears and worries themselves, or who protect their child from potentially risky experiences, will train their child to carry more fears than necessary. Anxiety is transferred to the child by this kind of display. Read books and stories to your child about children who have experienced similar fears. This helps children to talk about their fears and to find ways to cope.
- As with all emotions, fears become less of a problem for children as they gain self-confidence, see their world as a safe place, and find that fear is normal and can be dealt with.
- Some fears are normal and even helpful. But too many fears and anxieties can get in the way of enjoying everyday things such as learning in school, playing with a friend. That is the time when help is needed. You should take the child to a doctor who can help find out if a medical problem is making the child feel anxious. He can help find a way to lessen the anxiety through talking, relaxation exercises, medication or a combination of these activities.
- Parents have to be very patient while dealing with separation anxiety in their children. If they plan to go away for a few days leaving their child in someone else's care, they should give the child enough time to get accustomed to the new person. It has been observed that children who are used to being around different people right from a young age tend to be more independent and outgoing. Over-protective children are likely to be timid and withdrawn.

Temper tantrums

What are temper tantrums?

When children feel frustrated, angry or disappointed, they often express themselves by crying, screaming, breaking things, rolling on the floor, whining, holding their breath, kicking or hitting. Parents may feel angry, helpless or embarrassed at such behaviour. Temper tantrums are a normal part of a child's development as he learns self-control. In fact, all children have tantrums between the ages of 1 and 3. It is seen that by age 4, tantrums usually stop.

What is the cause?

Tantrums are not due to any physical or genetic cause but generally occur in those children who are pampered or spoilt. Sometimes the parents might not have enough time to spend with the child and tend to over compensate with toys and other gifts. This is particularly so in case of an only child. Temper tantrums are a way for a child to let off 'steam' when he is upset. Some other reasons for tantrums are that he may:

- Try to gain attention through tantrums
- Not fully understand what a parent is saying or asking, and may get confused
- Become upset when others cannot understand what he is saying
- Not have the words to describe his feelings and needs
- Have an illness or other physical problem that keeps him from expressing how he feels
- Be hungry but not recognize it
- Be tired or not getting enough sleep
- Be anxious and uncomfortable
- Not yet be able to do the things, such as walking and running, climbing down stairs or from furniture, drawing things, or making toys work
- Get irritable if he is not allowed to do what he wants to do.

How can these tantrums be prevented?

Children feel safe showing their feelings to the people they trust, hence they show more tantrums only in front of their parents. The following may help reduce the chances of a tantrum:

- Set reasonable limits and do not expect a child to be perfect. Give simple reasons for the rules you set, and don't change the rules.
- Keep a daily routine as much as possible, so that the child knows what to expect.
- Avoid situations that will frustrate the child, such as playing with children or toys that are too advanced for his abilities.

- Avoid outings or visits where the child has to sit still or cannot play for long periods of time.
- Meet the child's physical needs and give him adequate attention.
- Make sure that the child is well rested, especially before a busy day or stressful activity.
- Distract the child from activities likely to lead to a tantrum. Suggest different activities. Sometimes, something as simple as changing the location can prevent a tantrum.
- Set a good example. Avoid arguing or shouting in front of your child and lead by example by handling your own temper.
- Avoid excessive demands or restrictions.

Managing temper tantrums

Parents can sometimes tell when tantrums are coming. The child may seem moody, cranky or difficult. He may start to cry, kick, scream, fall to the ground or hold his breath. At other times, a tantrum may come on suddenly for no obvious reason. When the child has a temper tantrum, the suggestions below can help both the child and the parents get through it successfully.

1. Distract the child by calling his attention to something else, such as a new activity, book or toy. Sometimes just touching or stroking a child will calm him. You may need to gently restrain or hold the child. Interrupt his behaviour with a light comment like, 'I think there is a dog outside'. Humour or something as simple as a funny face can also help.
2. Try to remain calm. If you shout or become angry, it is likely to make things worse. Remember, the more attention you give to his behaviour, the more likely it is to happen again.
3. Minor displays of anger such as crying, screaming or kicking can usually be ignored. Stand nearby or hold the child without talking until he calms down.
4. Some temper tantrums cannot be ignored. The following kinds of behaviour should not be ignored and are not acceptable:

    - hitting or kicking parents or others
    - throwing things in a dangerous way
    - prolonged screaming or yelling.

5. If you cannot stay calm, leave the room. Wait a minute or two, or until his crying stops, before returning. Then help him get interested in something else. If the child is old enough, talk about what happened and discuss other ways to deal with it next time.
6. You should never punish the child for temper tantrums. He may start

to keep his anger or frustration inside, which can be unhealthy. Your response to tantrums should be calm and understanding.

7. Do not give a reward to the child for stopping a tantrum. Rewards may teach the child that a temper tantrum will help him get his way. When tantrums do not accomplish anything for the child, they are less likely to continue.
8. When the outbursts are severe or happen too often, they may be an early sign of emotional problems. Talk to a paediatrician if the child causes harm to himself or others during tantrums, for example if he holds his breath and faints, or if the tantrums get worse after the age of 4. The paediatrician will make sure that there are no serious physical or psychological problems causing the tantrums. He can also give you advise to help you deal with these outbursts.

It is important to realize that temper tantrums are a normal part of growing up. Tantrums are not easy to deal with but a loving, understanding and consistent approach will help a child through this part of his development. (*See also* page 100)

Sex education

The growth of your child into adolescence may put your parenting and communication skills to the test. Sex education varies according to the beliefs of a particular community. It depends on many factors - religious, cultural, economic and social.

Many consider that sex is something private and personal and should not be discussed in public. But these days, growing awareness on the prevention of AIDS and the use of condoms, has brought the discussion of sex into the open. You cannot avoid telling your child about sex these days. Even for the mental health and adjustment of your child, it is necessary to frankly tell him the facts of life when he asks questions about sex.

How to deal with children between the ages two and four?
During this period the child asks questions about the world around him and he will also ask about matters relating to differences between a boy and a girl. His genitalia are the same to him as his nose or fingers. He does not attribute any special function to them. Do not dodge his questions or refuse to answer, for then he will think there is something secretive about it. In any case he will find out as he grows older, so it is much better for him to hear about it from his parents.

A question like 'where do babies come from?' should obviously be answered in different ways to a 4-year-old and a 14-year-old. Answer the questions simply and say only as much as he can understand. Always tell the truth. However, you should not try to cover the whole field of sex in your answer, but just enough to satisfy his curiosity at that time. The process of birth is complicated enough for a child, so do not confuse him further. Having a pet in the house helps; you can discuss the question of puppies and kittens with him.

Sometimes he may ask the same question twice. Parents may think he is getting obsessed with sex. The simple reason is that he has forgotten the answers and he wants to ask the question again. Even when he is satisfied with your answers, he may come back later with more questions.

When does he become aware about himself?
Around the age of 3 years, a child becomes aware that he is a boy or she is a girl. He becomes aware that he has something extra, which his sister does not have. Similarly, a girl is aware that she lacks the appendage, which her brother has. Tell them that there is a difference, and to reassure

them, tell them the boy will grow up like his father and the girl like her mother.

How can you help them deal with sexuality?
From 2 or 3 years onwards, the child will explore his genitals just as he explores his mouth, nose and other parts of his body. Many parents get embarrassed and concerned about this. Do not threaten the child or slap him or laugh. This can be very disturbing to a child. It arouses fear and guilt and may make him feel that, in some way, that part of his body is dirty.

Some parents think that excessive handling of the male organs is, perhaps, due to his prepuce (skin covering the penis) irritating the child and they have him circumcised. The exploration of sex parts is normal for a child and nothing to be alarmed about. You can, however, give him plenty to do with his hands. Give him toys to play with and direct his attention elsewhere. Every time a child is naked, do not tease him. This attitude makes him terribly conscious of his sex. Privacy should be respected. These attitude carry on in adult life and may create psycho-sexual problems.

In fact, you need to worry if the child does not ask questions about sex. It may mean that his normal curiosity has somehow been curbed and he is resorting to friends, relatives, books or advertisements for information. He may, in the process, pick up information that is incorrect. In some schools, sex education is part of the curriculum. It is best that matters of sex are discussed with the child by parents or some senior member of the family with whom the child relates comfortably.

Your adolescent child needs to be given correct information about sex. Tell your daughter about menstruation before it happens. Similarly, tell your son about nocturnal emissions (wet dreams). Explain to the boy that nature provides an excess of seminal fluid and that it is perfectly normal, and to the girl that menstruation is nature's way of disposing of the unfertilized eggs.

You need to realize the importance of talking to your children. There may be very few teenagers who will directly ask their parents questions about sex. Emotional maturity at this age is rare and not expected of adolescents. Weaving discussions of sexual topics into everyday conversations – television shows, articles in books – may help your child consider sex as a normal part of life.

What is masturbation?
Sometimes small children of 2–4 years of age rub their thighs or play with their sex organs and find a pleasurable sensation accompanied by flushing of the face. This is known as masturbation. Like thumb-sucking, this will also stop as the child develops other interests. Distract him, but do not scold him or beat him. Masturbation is also common among adolescents. It is not the physical act itself that is unhealthy but the guilt which accompanies it. Give your child plenty of affection, make him feel wanted and needed, and once he is well occupied he may stop masturbating. The more satisfaction he gets from activities within and outside the home, the less he will want to masturbate.

Parents as well as children need to know that masturbation is a natural and harmless way of feeling sexual pleasure and of relieving sexual tension. You should try to answer your child's direct or indirect questions helping your child develop an informed and positive attitude towards sex and sexuality.

Fussy eaters

Every parent knows it is difficult to get children to eat nutritious food, whether it is a toddler who wants nothing but instant noodles or a teenager who lives on junk food and soft drinks. Children need to eat frequently to sustain their high energy levels and provide for their growing bodies.

Many young children go through periods of being fussy eaters and this is a normal part of growing up. Children often want to eat certain foods at a certain time and in a certain way. Many children, especially those from 18 months to 5 years of age are sometimes picky eaters. They eat what appears to an adult as a small amount of food, and yet they are well, active and growing normally. The term 'fussy eaters' is not used for children who are breastfeeding, but only for toddlers and children.

Some babies are very fussy while feeding, while others tend to doze off after a few minutes of feeding. The mother is not sure whether or not he has had his fill. But no sooner does she put him in the cot that he is up again and crying for feed.

What is the cause?

It may be that while feeding he is not in a comfortable position, or his nose is blocked due to secretions or being pushed against the breast. In a bottle-fed baby, the hole in the nipple may be so small that the child tires easily.

Fussy eating habits are generally acquired. An anxious mother is more likely to unknowingly encourage fussy eating habits. Making mealtimes a battleground can worsen the situation. Often there may be no obvious reason. The child's nervous system may not have matured enough to realize when his stomach is full. Whatever the reason, it makes the mother tense, which, in turn makes feeding even more difficult. The mother gets frustrated having to feed the child every half an hour, and the child remains unsatisfied and irritable. It is a vicious cycle.

What should parents do if their child does not appear healthy and growing normally?

In such a situation, it is important for the mother to remain calm and comforting towards the child. Shift him from one breast to the other. If he still goes to sleep, put him back in the cot very gently. If he cries soon after, try to comfort him. Maybe you can give him a few spoons of water to pacify him. Sometimes nothing works and you just have to be patient until the child quietens down.

If a child is a fussy eater and does not appear to be healthy or growing normally, parents should take the child to a physician for assessment. A child should never be forced to eat a specific food. However, if a child is hungry and is given a choice of foods, he is more likely to eat something. It is the role of parents to ensure that the foods from which a child can choose are all nutritious and appealing.

How should parents encourage their child to eat?

We all know that a healthy, varied diet is important for our child's growing needs. But what should you do if your child turns up his nose at just about everything.

Offer your child a wide variety of food – he will get a balanced diet. It is better for him to eat something that he likes even if you disapprove of it than to eat nothing at all.

If your child refuses to eat fruits and vegetables, try to make them more tempting or more fun, but do not camouflage a detested food by mixing it with something else. The child should eat because he wants to and not for any other reason. Encourage your child to feed himself.

- Serve food that is fresh and presented in an attractive way.
- Make mealtimes pleasant and relaxing.
- Talk about food; this may encourage a child to eat. Whenever possible, allow children to choose from one or two items on the menu (for example, a choice of peas or carrots for vegetables).
- Give your child the same food you eat.

You should be careful that the child is not overweight. Overweight children are more likely to become overweight adults. This can lead to many health problems.

Your child should eat a balanced diet. Start by setting a good example. If other members of your family commonly eat lots of fruits, vegetables, whole grains and low-fat dairy products, your kids will learn to eat a good diet. Kids tend to copy their parents, so if you eat well, they are more likely to eat well too. Do not get angry and do not panic if the child refuses to eat. If you are concerned about your child's dietary intake, talk to your doctor or a dietician. Put less on your child's plate and praise your child for eating even a little. Try to make meals enjoyable and not just about eating. Drinking too much liquid can lessen your child's appetite. Limit snacks and drinks between meals. This will help ensure that your child is hungry enough to eat solid foods. Do not overfeed. Obesity in children is rarely recognized by parents and is a major health problem.

Children's tastes change. One day they will hate something and a month later they'll love it. Fussy eaters are often slow eaters who dawdle over their plate. It is pointless trying to hurry them. Do not lose your cool at dinner. Simply remove the uneaten food.

If you find that these techniques are not working, there are people who can help. A registered dietician who specializes in children's nutritional needs can assess your situation and provide strategies for dealing with a picky eater.

Tips for coping with fussy eaters

- Try to serve meals that the rest of the family enjoys. Include one or two items that the fussy eater avoids, they may eat the items while watching others enjoy them.
- Try to serve smaller portions of food to your child.
- Invite a friend of the child who eats well. This sometimes works well.
- Invite for dinner an adult that the child likes such as an uncle or friend. Sometimes a child will eat in the company of someone else without any fuss.
- If your child is playing with his food, quietly remove the plate without any fuss.
- Make mealtimes enjoyable and talk about what the child is doing.
- Limit snacks and drinks between meals so the child feels hungrier at mealtimes.
- Offer drinks after a meal so that they don't ruin the appetite.
- Offer new foods when you know your child is hungry and more receptive to new tastes.
- Do not substitute milk for meals.

Speech disorders

Speech is a component of language by which humans communicate with each other through spoken words. Language also has other components, which aid communication but are not verbal in nature.

The most important period for normal speech development in humans is the first 3 years of life. This is the time when the brain is maturing and is at its receptive best and can be maximally stimulated for talking. This is known as the 'critical period' for speech acquisition.

The infant begins by crying for food or when he is uncomfortable. By around 2 months of age, the infant starts cooing which is a repetitive sound consisting only of vowels. By 6 months, the baby starts to combine vowels and consonants to produce sounds like 'baaa-baaa', which is called babbling. By the end of the first year, most children are able to say a few simple words like 'dada'. This ability to speak enhances by the end of the second year, where a child is able to combine two words to communicate his wishes. Though these are the broad milestones for speech development, speech development varies with individual children. Speech disorders refer to difficulties in producing speech sounds or problems with voice quality. There may be a problem with the flow of words (stuttering), unclear production of speech, or problem with the volume and pitch of voice. There may also be trouble in using certain speech sounds like substitution of 'f' with 's' (lisping). The child may also have the problem of limited speech where he may not talk at all or may have trouble talking in specific situations.

Parents are usually the first to notice the disorder in the child. A paediatrician may then diagnose the problem after taking the child's medical history and a physical examination. A hearing test may be done to rule out deafness as a possible cause. Other tests like a CT scan may be ordered to examine any nervous system damage. In cases where a psychological disturbance is suspected, the child may be referred to a child psychologist for confirmation of the condition.

The treatment depends on the cause. In children who have a physical defect, an operation may have to be done to correct the problem. In children with hearing impairment, a hearing aid is fitted and speech therapy is started as soon as possible. For all children, speech therapy is done in addition to the medical or surgical treatment. Speech therapy helps to clear the child's diction, pitch and tone of voice or stuttering.
(*See also* page 174)

Stammering ... and how to overcome it

There are more than 45 million people in the world today who stammer and approximately 10 million live in India. Stammering is predominantly a 'male' condition (80% of all stammerers are male) and it usually affects the first-born male child. The majority of stammerers (65%) have a family history of the disorder; usually the father who stammers or speaks at a rapid rate. Nearly always, stammering starts before the child is 5 years of age. If left untreated, it peaks in severity around the age of 10 to 18 years and then begins to stabilize or fade away as the stammerer grows older.

A stammerer knows precisely what he wants to say but cannot, for the moment, say it because of an involuntary repetition, prolongation or cessation of the speech sound. Research suggests that the disorder might be caused due to a 'neurological mistiming' during the act of speech which leaves the stammerer confused about when exactly to say the word he wants to say. Speaking is not merely the movement of the tongue but involves a fine coordination of both mental and physical processes. Like all other physical actions, the act of speech is the result of neuro-muscular coordination which involves the transmitting of electrochemical messages from the brain to the appropriate muscle groups. For everyone of us (non-stammerers and stammerers alike), this neuro-muscular system sometimes trips and fails especially during moments of inadequate emotional control. For the stammerer, this 'tripping' occurs much more frequently than it does for normal speakers. Whenever he faces what he perceives as a 'feared' situation, the stammerer adopts a mind-set which triggers off spasms of speech-blocks. Such fears can also centre around certain speech sounds or even certain people.

Actually, all stammerers have periods of fluency when they are emotionally relaxed but revert back to dysfluent speech under stress. Answering the roll call in class, speaking on the telephone, talking to someone in authority, speaking in a group, attending a job interview, etc., are some such pressure situations which might cause an increase in stammering behaviour.

One more unusual fact about stammering is that even the severest stammerer can sing fluently without any speech blocks. This is because when we sing a song, we know exactly when to say the words and there is no ambiguity in our minds about their timing. In conversational speech, however, we cannot bank on any such cues. As normally fluent speakers, most of us do not need these cues. However, without these cues, a stammerer's speech becomes disoriented, because of his 'wrongly tuned' neurological speech-timing system. He experiences difficulty in maintaining a smooth flow of words in the sentences he speaks. Frequently repeated, these instances of stammering arouse fear in the mind of the child who stammers. With growing years, these fears keep snowballing until the stammerer begins to experience tremendous frustration, anxiety, shame, embarrassment, even guilt every time he opens his mouth to speak. He begins to recoil from speaking. The smirks on the faces of his listeners which his speech sometimes elicits do nothing to help his self-confidence. In every other respect, except speaking ability, the stammerer is a completely normal human being, as good or bad as the rest of us. In fact most stammerers are sensitive and intelligent people.

Some psychiatrists might prescribe tranquillizers in the belief that relieving stress would help speech fluency. Such drugs usually complicate, rather than resolve the issue and are strongly discouraged for the treatment of stammering by most speech pathologists.

Hypnosis has also shown unpromising results in the treatment of stammering. A few stammerers who might become fluent while under a trance invariably return to stammering when out of the hypnotic state. Yoga and meditation might really hold the key to solving the problem of stammering. With the greater sense of emotional and intellectual balance that these disciplines promote, the stammerer might find them of tremendous help in his attempts to develop better control over his speech.

These are aspects that can be changed through self-therapy to help the person overcome his speaking difficulty. Speech is one of our body's strongest habits and stammered speech is also a habit. Stammering is not a disease and, therefore, it cannot be treated through medicines. The stammering child or adult has to be helped to develop a new, more fluent manner of speech through an intensive reorientation programme which focuses on modifying his physical manner of talking as well as changing his mental attitude towards the problem.

Many of us might experience a feeling of embarrassment when we converse with stammerers; some of us look away while others go ahead to complete their sentences for them. In talking with a stammerer, the following hints might be of help.

- Listen to what is said, not how it is said.
- Be patient and don't hurry the person talking.
- Try to maintain natural eye contact.
- Simplistic advice ('breathe properly', 'don't worry', 'don't be afraid', etc.) though well-meant is not always helpful.

- Stammerers have difficulty when talking but don't assume they are stupid or confused about what they are saying.
- Many stammerers have difficulty when they speak on the telephone. Please do not hang up if the caller is taking longer than usual or if he is silent for a while.

Stammerers usually try and hide their speech problem from their listeners. This attempt at camouflage is counter-productive because it only acts as psychological 'fuel' for even more speech-blocks. If the stammerer is open about his speech difficulty, he experiences lesser stress and is able to speak with greater control.

In the final analysis, stammering can be overcome if the sufferer seeks scientific, professional guidance and is ready to work towards achieving speech fluency through regular practice of therapeutic techniques. It certainly cannot disappear by ingesting some magic potent!

Difficult children

28. Why does my niece keep crying for small things?

Q. My niece is 5 years old with a one-and-a-half-year-old brother. She is a loving, soft, kind-hearted and a brilliant child with very good academic and extracurricular skills. She loves to play like other children of her age and is an extrovert. However, several traits in her need improvement; the most common being crying. She is very timid and afraid of the dark. She's also afraid of some toys such as a radio-controlled car. She has attended 10 swimming classes but doesn't go beyond drenching her feet. She cries a lot when she doesn't find her toys. Yet, she doesn't attempt to search for them, instead she starts crying. The funny part is that she won't accept that she has seen the object she was searching for. Ignoring her crying for these things helps. But we want to cultivate independence in her. She doesn't want wrong things to be pointed out. While doing her maths homework, if we find faults with her calculations, she starts crying and denies it being wrong. If we point out a wrong note being played on the piano, she starts crying. She doesn't try anything new. This quality can pose a big problem as it lowers her confidence. The idea that she might do something wrong, inhibits her from trying. While playing hide and seek with her friend, if she doesn't find her in a few minutes, she gets scared and starts crying. It is tough to get her to do something, as it needs much pampering. At school, when the teacher distributes question papers to students one by one, she fears that she might not get one and starts crying if she's not the first one to get it. My sister and brother-in-law are well educated and ensure that they spend ample time with her. They are very encouraging, supportive, patient and communicative and give her all the attention she needs. Yet, she craves for more and ends up crying to achieve the same. Please advise.

A. You seem to be an observant and caring uncle! You have sent a very detailed observation of your niece. She does seem more sensitive and vulnerable than normal children. Perhaps her condition started or has been aggravated with the birth of her brother. Sometimes children, who have a new sibling, feel scared that they will no longer have a place in the parents' affection. One just has to reassure her about that and keep some time only for her.

As you suggest, ignoring her crying helps, but is not always possible. Distracting her at that times could be tried. But, more importantly, you will have to develop ways of rewarding her for not crying. Make it a game. Increase the hours of 'no crying' gradually. Explain that if she does not cry at all during the day, some treat will be given (something she likes to do) before she sleeps. Play soft music, preferably classical, while she is winding down.

Ask her teachers how they discourage her crying – surely they find it difficult too. The child needs reassurance, but also a firm no-nonsense attitude, once you have assured her.

You say that her parents give her all the love she needs. But she seems to feel otherwise. I think that the child and the parents should sit down peacefully together and openly discuss the problem when they have unhurried time. Sometimes verbalization of a problem helps everyone to see it more clearly. Since the child is bright, surely she will follow the discussion and the pros and cons. I am also wondering if the girl feels that too much is expected of her (piano, maths, etc.). It would be better not to focus on her achievements, but to emphasize the fun and enjoyment she gets out of her activities. Let her play the piano, but don't rush in to point out each error. If she has an ear for music, she will realize it herself soon enough.

You have not mentioned her health or physical skills. Sometimes, children who are slightly built and low in weight can be pushed down by their playmates and may feel vulnerable. Make sure her protein intake is improved and that cola drinks are avoided.

Parents should be interested in the child even when she is not doing something specific. It is in the informal moments that most codes of behaviour are taught and learnt. All the best in your avuncular role!

29. How do I deal with a whimsical child?

Q. My daughter, 4-and-a-half years of age, is very bright and analytic. Academically, she is fast and perfect. But she is whimsical and anything she

does is only at her will. No one can convince or force her to do anything. She can narrate stories nicely and every time while narrating stories she can translate her dreams in an enjoyable form. She seems to concoct events according to her wishes. She can carry on with such things endlessly. Sometimes it appears she is lying. This puts her in trouble at home as well as outside, particularly in school. And as father, I fail to understand what exactly has happened. After one or two days we only have some idea of the actual event. Generally it is not that serious but she makes a big mess of it. She does not disclose the happening even to her mother; instead she makes stories. Some people say it is lying. Please advise.

A. Sometimes, children do not have a clear idea of the difference between reality and fantasy; that is, between what they see and what they imagine. It is a little confusing for them. However, this should not be treated as telling a lie.

You may have noticed that the events your child talks about are not necessarily to her benefit. For example, if a child takes a pencil that belongs to a friend and then claims that she got it as a present for a birthday from an uncle – that could be a lie. But if the child tells her friends that she had 20 friends over for an ice cream party, it is different from a lie. This is what is called wishful thinking. The story may reflect what the child would wish could happen. We read stories to the child that describe magical things and it is quite possible that she absorbs that kind of story and makes up her own. I have known many children who do this. If the children are bright and articulate, and if they feel that they are getting the attention of adults by their stories, they may add to the story. Without making a big issue of it, you could tell the child to let you know if what she just described 'really' happened or not. But do not use the term lying for her stories. Ask her if she made up the story. Enjoy it and laugh with her. But give even closer attention when something she actually experienced is the subject of her conversation.

In a well-known novel *Uncle Tom's Cabin*, a child found that whenever she confessed to taking something, she was praised and rewarded for owning up. So she kept on confessing to having taken things that she had not taken at all!

Children want your time and your approval. Maybe if you consciously spend more time with her doing things together, she may realize that it is not necessary to astonish you with a good story, to catch your attention. There are simple craft activities, such as vegetable printing and making sail boats out of paper, that can be done together. According to Madame Montessori, real life has enough excitement (ants, butterflies, lizards, the evening sky, for example) that very young children do not need fairy stories. Not all educators are agreed on this, but we have to suit the treatment to the child. In the Montessori system, asking the child to help with small tasks around the house is good. Even washing out handkerchiefs is a great activity for a 4-year-old.

Children outgrow most of these phases, but you are right to consider the matter, in order to avoid any future problem. (*See also* page 9)

30. How should we tackle our child's misbehaviour?

Q. My son is 3 years old. Since I am working, he goes to a day boarding school. Earlier he used to be with our maid the whole day. My son has developed a habit of spitting at everybody and he beats up people around him when we don't allow him to do what he wants to. Our maid used to call boys at home in our absence. So, sometimes my son follows their actions. We feel very shameful and are very tense about him. His teacher says that he is a well-behaved and an affectionate child. When we hit him, he cries like anything. Please suggest what should we do and how should we tackle him?

A. It is evident that your son is not getting enough positive parental attention. He has also been exposed to negative behaviours of the maid and her male friends. You should be glad that he is well behaved at school. To make sure that he gets warmth and appreciation at home, please follow the advice:

- Do not use physical punishment, as it generally has an undesirable impact.
- Give him quality time, love and encouragement for his desirable behaviour.
- Be good parental models yourselves.
- Try to divert his attention when he is about to spit or hit someone. Tell him firmly that such behaviour is not acceptable.
- If possible, enlist support of grandparents to provide him with a sense of security as well as supervision.

31. How should I handle my hypersensitive daughter?

Q. My daughter is 4 years old. We live in the USA. She has started going to school. She is very sensitive and considers all our suggestions as a scolding. We are not supposed to say anything even when she is at fault. Her teacher

said something to her in school, due to which she is not ready to go to school. She cries badly when we ask her to go to school. I have tried my level best to convince her softly and even physically. But she does not respond. She remained absent from school for the past one week. How should I handle my hypersensitive daughter?

A. Your daughter seems to be extremely sensitive and, to modify her behaviour, it is important to analyse if there is any modification required in the parents' behaviour and attitudes. Some children are inherently more sensitive, but usually it is the handling by parents that increases this emotional reactivity. Some steps that can be taken are:

- Convey to her that you disapprove of her action, but still love her unconditionally.
- Do not encourage her over-emotional behaviour. Try ignoring it. On the other hand, give her attention and encouragement when she shows positive behaviour.
- Be firm and consistent in disciplining. Do not change your stance if you or the other parent has said no to something, and she starts crying.
- Prove to be good role models yourselves.

32. Why does my son bite other children when he can't put forth his point of view?

Q. Both my husband and I are working parents of a 4-year-old son. Our son has a problem of biting people when he can't put across his point of view. At times, it becomes difficult for him to play with his friends or cousins. We thought this behaviour was due to our absence from home, feeling of insecurity which he was unable to convey. Therefore, we shifted him to his grandmother's care. There he has a 5-and-a-half year old cousin to play and communicate with. But he still bites his cousin at times. He also has a bedwetting problem and even wets his pants. He is a poor eater as well. How can we change his habits?

A. I think your son is rather disturbed. You need to take him to a child psychiatrist, if one is available in the city where you live. If such a person cannot be found, you must consult some expert to identify the problem. It is not a simple case of changing his habits. We will have to work with restoring his confidence in himself and in the setting in which he finds himself.

His grandmother may also find it difficult to look after him. If it is possible for the mother of the child to spend less time away, it might begin to restore the child's sense of security. If that cannot be done immediately, just a lot of hugging and cuddling and show of affection will be necessary. Biting is his method to convey the message that he does not appreciate his circumstances!

When he sees you, does he express some joy? Does he cry when you leave him? Even these would be positive signs. Please do discuss this with helpful family members and friends and do what is best for the child. A continuation of the present setting will not help, in my view.

33. How should I handle a demanding and rash child?

Q. My son is 4-and-a-half years old. He is an above average child as per his teachers. He is very imaginative and restless. He talks too much, is very authoritative and hits one and all. I am a working woman and he stays with his grandparents. They are aggressive and stubborn. They start fighting and shouting at the slightest provocation. They generally cater to all his demands whether justified or unjustified. My son is very demanding, rash in temperament and answers back, using the worst words when retaliating. I am a loving and firm mother to him. I cannot do much to change the habits of my in-laws. They are not receptive to any ideas proposed by me and are easily offended no matter how polite I am. My husband tours a lot and is seldom available for help. I am unable to discipline my child and am anxious about his personality development. He is good at dramatics and has an ear for music too. He is especially good with numbers.

A. Your son's world is too small for him. In other words, he has the energy and inclination for many more activities. Perhaps you should get him started on special classes for music or drama. Let him join a club, where he has to cope with mental and physical challenges. When all his demands are met at home, he is being reinforced for making more demands. Since you leave him with grandparents, it is likely that he will imitate what he sees and hears.

If the city you live in has an after-school daycare arrangement, you should look into the possibilities for your child. Also, consider if you can adjust your working hours so that you have more time with the child. The child's father should also take an active role in the child's socialization. The number of hours he spends with his son is not as important as what activities he plans and how they communicate when they are together. Consult your son's teacher at school and see if you can work together to reduce the child's aggression.

Alongside, please cut down the hours of his TV watching and cut out cola drinks from his diet. Both are known to be harmful.

34. How can I handle my son's short attention span?

Q. My 3-year-old son started going to school 2 months back. The teachers have been telling me that it is very difficult to get him to sit in one place. Also, it is difficult to make him do certain activities such as painting, sticking, etc. He cannot sit still. How can this be handled? Is he hyperactive or is his attention or interest in things short-lived? Please advise.

A. Many children, especially boys, like to move around and not sit in one place for long. Our preschool centres are not always equipped to handle such active children. He is not 'hyperactive', though the term is used by many to mean 'very active'. Please note that all children are not exactly alike and at 3 years of age, all of them have a short attention span.

The best thing for you to do would be to plan at least half an hour of vigorous activity for him. Let him do a lot of running around and jumping before he goes to school, so that he feels inclined to take part in the quieter activities that the school provides.

35. How should we manage our son who is very naughty?

Q. I am residing in Dubai with my wife and a 3-year-old son for the past 7 years. Every year, we all go for a vacation for a month to India. Since the beginning my son is very naughty and he hates to eat food, but now he has become very destructive and he does not like to eat food. He just runs in the house and breaks all his toys and, if we stop him, he shouts back to us and he has hit his mother many a times. We sent him to kindergarten for one year and discussed the above problem with his teacher. She also said that many a time he screams but does listen to her and is fine in the classroom. Since the beginning, he was not eating food so we used to force feed him but now he does not allow us to do that also. When we go for shopping he starts running and throws things from the shelves and creates chaos if we try to stop him. We have punished him many a time by taking his best toys away or warning him that if he misbehaves, we will not take him to shopping malls

or the garden. For some time he is fine but again starts doing the same things. We tried everything possible but all in vain. Please suggest something.

A. Since your son seems to have adjusted to school, perhaps his problem can be managed with firm, consistent and quiet discipline. For the child to calm down, the excitement of television and visits to malls should be reduced. Concentrated foods (like nutritious malted milk) may be given, to assure that he gets at least a minimum amount of food in him. Soft drinks should be avoided, as the caffeine in cola drinks makes children more aggressive. As far as possible, do not give him many instructions at one time. Break up the information into bits that he can handle. Even if you are angry, do not raise your voice. Sounds may already be magnified for him and he needs quietness and clear instructions. When you come to India for your vacation, do consult an experienced psychologist or special educator about how to plan activities for your son. Doctors are often too busy with major medical issues, to give you time and advice. (*See also* page 9)

36. How do I deal with a jealous and aggressive child?

Q. My daughter is 5 years old. She feels extremely jealous when I appreciate others, especially her peers. Is this normal? At times she is aggressive? How should I deal with such behaviour?

A. It is very normal for children to feel jealous if parents give attention to another child. They usually outgrow this behaviour. The main problem comes when the child is a sibling. It is important for you to explain that you love her, but also find the other children likeable. It should be made very clear that aggression will not be allowed. Ignore her crying behaviour and appreciate her when she does not show aggression or jealousy. (*See also* pages 9, 100)

Habits

37. How can my child give up the habit of nail biting?

Q. My daughter is 4 years old and has been biting her nails and skin around it since the past six months. First it seemed to be just a bad habit, but it has gone from bad to worse with her doing it all the time. It has started affecting her diet too, she does not eat her dinner like she used to. I thought it was something she did more when she was shy, at some get-together but it is getting out of hand. My husband, his mum and his dad (deceased) all bite their nails. My husband says he does it as he thinks it is a nervous disposition and it is genetic since his father's brother and sister do it too. He thinks that my daughter has inherited this nervous disposition and hence we need to treat it medically. My husband suffers from colitis (stomach disorder) and though nail biting has not been its sole cause, it has contributed towards it, according to him. I want to find out what is the psychological and physical cause behind this habit? What can I do to help my daughter discontinue this habit before it is too late? She is enthusiastic and full of life in her nursery, leading her friends etc., but in new surroundings, she takes time to settle in and is very shy and apprehensive. She starts school 3 months from now and is petrified of spiders and flies. I am hopeful that you will help me find a solution to help her and make her give up the habit in time before she starts full-time education.

A. To begin with, there is no known gene for nail biting. However, it is possible that the tendency to get anxious could be passed from father to child. It seems to me that your child's nail biting should be tackled in three or four different ways. If her father or other adults around her have the bad habit, she can pick it up just by imitation. So the first thing would be for them to avoid it. On the face of it, this would not be easy. You must explain to her that the habit would put off her friends from getting close to her or playing games with her. When she listens to you and avoids nail biting for even one hour at a time, you can give her a small reward. If she gives in to her habit, tell her that you will have to withdraw some privilege (such as watching cartoons on TV or listening to a bedtime story). Increase the praise and the rewards, if she remains strong-willed and resists nail biting.

In the old days, mothers and grandmothers would put some neem oil on the finger being sucked. The unpleasant taste would be associated in the child's mind with the behaviour. Gradually, she would give it up. It is very natural for her to be a little shy in a new situation. But you must convince her that instead of biting her nails, there are other ways of handling it. She could tell herself that it is all right and that she won't be scared. If you teach her some little prayer, she could silently say it to herself, in a new situation and the worst few seconds would be over. It is also necessary to be with her at bedtime and to dispel her fears. No child is normally fond of spiders or flies, but there is no reason to be petrified of them. Perhaps, she has had some experience in her infancy, which has left some fear in her, but all conditions can be treated, with affection and a common sense approach. For example, the song familiar to most preschoolers, 'Eensy-weensie spider' makes the spider playful and nice to watch. She could get over her fear of spiders in a month or two by singing that song and making drawings of spiders. Talk to the child and listen to her carefully.

The important thing is to find out why she is anxious. Make sure that the servants in the house or neighbours who drop in have not said or done something to upset her. Let her play with 4 or 5 dolls and make up her own stories about them. Sometimes children will make the dolls go through what they are experiencing. If you observe quietly, you may be able to locate her reasons for being anxious. Do all this in a gentle, friendly and affectionate way and never with anger. Do not hit or punish her to get her to obey you. Take the child as a partner in this effort. Don't make the beginning of formal school the time marker for all her behaviours. Otherwise, starting school could become something that she would be worried about. In any case, she should give up the practice of nail biting, which is only a reflection of an anxiety that she cannot talk about. Time, patience and love will make the best combination for the treatment. (*See also* page 9)

School issues

38. Can study overload at preschool level affect the child's health?

Q. Nowadays, children at lower kindergarten (LKG) and upper kindergarten (UKG) level (4–6 years) are overloaded. If the input is more at this level, will it have any effect on their health in general after 10 or 15 years?

A. Overloading the child with studies and having undue expectations at the elementary school stage can result in physical and psychological stress. Since the child may not be able to deal with the pressure, she may get a sense of failure and hence suffer from low self-esteem. A negative attitude towards school and studies is also possible. These consequences could have long-term undesirable effects on physical and mental health. But the people who run children's schools seem unaware of all this. Parents seem to have very little choice in the matter. If you do have a choice, shift your child to a system that has more play and less curricular load. Children do have a great deal of resilience and seem to survive bad schooling!

39. How can I deal with a child who refuses to go to school?

Q. My 4-year-old daughter has just joined preschool. She went to school happily for the first week, but now she starts crying when we ask her to go to school. She is very sensitive. As such nothing has happened in her school. We tried our level best to convince her politely and patiently. At last we had to handle her physically and sent her to school forcefully. But she started crying again the next day. How should I handle her? Should we be non-

cooperative to her at home or threaten her or wait till she changes her mind? I don't want to take any step that will affect her future. How can I make her strong-minded, and less sensitive?

A. Most children go through this phase of crying while going to school, but it is better that the child is dealt with firmly yet lovingly. You have to convey your messages of affection and security, both verbally and non-verbally.

- Reassure her of the fact that you love her very much and this is a temporary separation, which is necessary for her education and future.
- Give her a signal that her crying will not always result in her demands being met – in this context, not wanting to go to school.
- Share with her how nice it is to grow up and how much fun going to school is, so that she acquires positive attitudes towards school. These signals will definitely help her adjust to going to school. The parents could also perhaps introduce her to other preschoolers from the family or neighbourhood.

40. At what age should a child start writing?

Q. What is the correct age to make a child write/scribble (alphabets/ numbers/drawing, etc.) in a notebook or slate? Most of the schools in this city insist on making a child write even when he joins a playgroup or nursery.

A. A child is not psychologically ready to read or write before the age of 5 years, but there are large individual differences. The best option is to understand your own child's readiness level and give suitable opportunities. Forcing a child who is not ready can lead to problems. But nursery schools do seem to do a 'fast forward' and parents are left without a choice. I wish teachers who run playschools would also write in to us with their doubts, but they appear to be riding on absolute certainty. Ultimately, one finds that the children are resilient and cope with everything!

41. Why doesn't my son respond to attendance in the class?

Q. My younger son is 4 years old. Due to his health problems, our social gatherings had to stop. He is a shy boy and never used to speak with his playschool teacher. Even at home, if we ask him to recite a poem he will

recite it only if we do not keep an eye contact with him. Now he is in nursery. His teacher told us that he is very talkative among his friends but when she calls for attendance he doesn't respond. She even punished him by making him stand facing the wall and told him that he can sit only if he says 'Yes Madam!' in response to the roll call. He started rolling on the floor and crying. He behaves this way at home also, when someone insists him on doing something. Earlier, we thought that he is an introvert, but his teacher says he is not introvert but adamant. His elder brother is 8 years old and is an extrovert and social child. How can we change our younger son's behaviour?

A. Each child is unique, with different ways of doing things and with different levels of self-confidence and sociability. Stop comparing your two sons.

Some children are very strong-willed and hate to be under anyone's control. When the teacher punished your son and humiliated him in front of the whole class, he was upset. The teacher can also develop other ways of taking attendance, but you cannot tell her that.

There is no formula for changing behaviour. Persuasion is the best method. A little humour, while dealing with a tricky problem will lead to its solution. We are all too earnest about obedience and good behaviour and too unforgiving of individuality and unconventionality.

If your child is shy, do not force him to be outgoing. Let him develop at his own pace.

42. My child is unable to write properly, what should I do?

Q. I have a 4-year-old son who goes to school and is in KG. I send him for extra classes but the only problem with him is that he uses his left hand to write, which is making it very tough for him to hold the pencil tightly and write. He is very smart and knows all his school poems. Can you please suggest what should I do? When he was 3-and-a-half years old, I admitted him to an English-medium school and he was there for only 3 months. The teachers started complaining that he does not respond and when forced, he vomits. Then I shifted him to an Indian school where the teacher complains that he can only write with the help of dots. He has started writing the alphabet A, but writing B is a problem.

A. I am glad you shifted your son out of a school that forced him to write at age 3 and forced him to the point of making him vomit.

If your son has a tendency to be left-handed, it is best to let him develop that. Let him use the left hand for writing, throwing a ball or picking up something. If you force him to become right-handed, he may develop speech problems at a later time. It is probably not because he uses his left hand that he is slow. Expecting all 4-year-old children to write the alphabet is unrealistic. But he has to adjust to the school you send him to!

How can we tell the teachers what to do? Perhaps you should try talking to the teacher and asking if your child can continue dotted alphabets for a bit longer, as a special case of being a left-hander.

Give him plenty of activities at home such as drawing on the floor with chalk, using crayons to draw or colour and playing with sand, clay and water. It may be messy for you to clean up, but those are the activities that will help his eye–hand coordination and his fine muscle development. An added advantage is that such activities are also enjoyable.

Once in a while, while making chapatis, give him some dough to play with and to shape the atta as he likes. Let him also roll out the dough and make a small chapati for you! There are many other methods which are used in good nursery schools. For instance, you can draw a circle or triangle and ask the child to put pebbles (small stones or tamarind seeds) on the shape. The same can be done with letters and numbers, to make the child familiar with them. Having the child use a rope and tie simple knots or learn to lace shoes and turn socks inside out – anyone of these everyday tasks will help his muscular development. Use music and rhythmic movements for added joy!

Watch your child and give him things to do, which he can do well. New things can be introduced gradually. Do not be angry at what he cannot do, but learn to appreciate what he can. You will find much difference. (*See also* page 116)

43. My child is brilliant but does not talk in school, what should we do?

Q. My daughter is 3 years and 4 months old. She is very talented and can identify big and small letters; can write them and also write and say the numbers from 1–30. She loves puzzles, educational toys, CDs, etc., and has been using the computer to work on educational CD from the age of 2-and-a-half years. She knows lots of rhymes and in my opinion is an above average student. I joined her in pre-KG class for 2 months and this year she is going to LKG. She comes and narrates everything at home and is up to date in her lessons. The problem is she is not communicating with her teacher. She writes and shows everything on the slate, but just nods to answer questions

as 'yes' or 'no' and refuses to talk to the teacher even though she knows the lessons. Right now the exams are going on. She just wrote the written part but refused to say the oral part. I have tried asking if she doesn't like the teacher but she says she likes the teacher but she can't speak in school and becomes tongue-tied, whereas at home she takes all her dolls and playacts school and the teacher. She comes home and teaches us the stuff her teacher has taught her with all the actions. What can I do to help her speak up and gain her confidence? She is an only child as my elder son died due to SIDS when he was 6 months old. I have taught her to the best of my ability and she also learns eagerly. She is very much interested in books. How can she get over being tongue-tied at school? She says she will talk to the teacher but at school she gets stuck and no words comes out. Please advise.

A. Let me congratulate you on having a brilliant child. She is not just above average; she is way ahead of others at her age. Her achievements are exceptional. Why don't you let her gradually get over her shyness to speak up in class? Even the teacher must realize that the child has learnt what is taught in class. Forcing her to speak and making a lot of fuss about her shyness is not going to help her. I know many persons who were shy as children, but have become outgoing adults. We cannot expect all children to be in the same mould. As long as the child is playing, learning, eating and sleeping well and relates to her parents, she is doing 'fine'. One of these days she will start talking in class and in response to the teacher's questions. I really do not think that there is anything you can do. Self-confidence, especially in a public sphere like the school, develops slowly in case of some children. More than anything else, we have to accept that each child is unique. We also know stories of athletes and sportspersons who were sickly in their childhood and have reached great heights later. Just relax and, if you can, request the teacher to help the child by not demanding a reply each time. By next year, she will be chattering away like everyone else. If her not speaking in class continues and is considered a problem by the school, write to me again, six months later. Meanwhile, enjoy the childhood of your talented child. (*See also* page 9)

44. Why doesn't my daughter mingle with her classmates?

Q. My daughter is 4 years and 8 months old. She is being promoted to UKG. She has been performing well in LKG, but her teacher complains that she

does not mingle with her classmates. She is very quiet in the class. According to her teacher, she is very responsive to all the questions. What should be done to make her mingle with her classmates?

A. Children have their own temperaments and we should not expect everyone to be in the same mould. Many children are shy in the beginning but open up gradually. Since your daughter is responsive in class, there should be no cause for worry. If your daughter is an only child at home surrounded by adults, she may not be used to interacting or sharing things with peers. Talk to her to find out what keeps her from interacting with her classmates. You can also try inviting some of her classmates to your home, maybe for a festival or for her birthday party. It might be fun for them to play simple games or sing together. That may break the ice. Above all, do not label her in any way, and do not force her to be sociable. Any change will come gradually. (*See also* page 9)

45. Why has my son lost his concentration in studies?

Q. My 4-and-a-half-year-old son is studying in lower primary. He has completed his pre-primary and first term of lower KG in Tamil Nadu. The school there was very strict and he was considered an outstanding student. Then we got transferred to our native state, where he joined a reputed school, which is not very strict in the primary level. For the first few weeks he was a very good student. He became very active as compared to his earlier school. Now his teacher complains that he is not at all attentive in the class and keeps talking and playing all the time. This causes disturbance to other students also. His teacher says that he is a very talented boy with a very good grasping power. But nowadays he is very playful and does not concentrate at all on what his teacher says. How can I handle this problem?

A. Your child is obviously not finding class work challenging enough and is, therefore, getting distracted. This can be a serious problem not only for the teachers and parents but also for the child himself. This happens in cases of children who are very intelligent.

You should try to keep in constant touch with his teacher. She needs to make special efforts at making him interested. She may need to be firm in discipline too. If possible you may consider shifting his section to get him into one where the majority are approximately at his level. A shift of school may also be considered. Children of 4 years of age need to be active and to have a variety of play materials. It is possible that his class work is dull. Talk to him patiently and work out a solution.

He may give you clues on whether he finds studies very easy or whether the teacher does not give enough attention. You could reason with him. Make him understand the value of getting the most out of his school experiences. Get him books, games and puzzles with which he can be happily engaged at home.

Fussy eaters

46. My child has no interest in food. What should I do?

Q. My 4-year-old son is normal in every respect. But I have problems in feeding him and it takes me at least an hour to feed him rice and dal. He keeps the food in his mouth for a long time. If I let him eat on his own, he makes a mess out of it. Most of the time he just plays with the food. If I wait for him to be hungry and ask for food, he becomes so hungry that he starts crying for milk and does not eat any food at all. The teacher at his preschool says that he does not eat snacks. Will it be a good idea to keep him in the company of other kids of his age for a few days so that he learns to eat on his own by seeing them? What other remedies can I try?

A. Eating problems are common in young children and are best addressed by not fussing over them. Do not give in to his demand for milk whenever he is hungry. Do not keep too many snacks or junk food handy. Instead keep fruits and vegetables around. Try and cook some special dishes for him, which are interesting in appearance and taste. Make mealtimes relaxed and not battlegrounds. It is definitely a good idea to let the child eat with other children. Make sure that he is de-wormed and has no infestation.

47. Why does my child take such a long time to eat food?

Q. My daughter is 5 years old. She eats very slowly and takes about an hour to chew one chapatti. I tell her stories, show her cartoons but daily she makes me shout. Everyday I have to tell her to eat faster and finish her food.

Till now she has never asked for food herself. I have tried lots of tricks, but there is no effect on her. A single bite remains in her mouth for hours and she eats so slowly that everyone gets irritated in the house. Kindly suggest me some remedy.

A. Some children have a genuine problem about swallowing. It is not necessarily being stubborn. You should consult a good paediatrician to ensure that she does not have a physiological problem. For some time, you could stop forcing her to eat chapatti and give her softly cooked food, such as rice or sooji or an interesting soup. An omelette will be a good addition to her diet. She needs to get enough nourishment. Shouting at her will not help anybody, least of all, your daughter. If she likes fruit, that could be added to her daily intake. She must have plenty of milk and milk products, such as butter, cheese and yogurt.

Make sure that you spend some of her playtime with her and that the adults she is fond of are available to her, other than at mealtimes. Often, children take a long time over their meals, because it is the time that the mother surely spends with them. I am not saying that it is so in every case. I am just helping you to identify the roots of her eating problem. Asking elders in the family may also help, as they would have dealt with similar issues.

Parenting

48. I am a working mother and my child doesn't listen to me. What should I do?

Q. My husband and I are working parents of a 4-and-a-half year-old daughter. She stays with my in-laws throughout the day. At the end of the day when we pick her up, we face a lot of adamancy and misbehaviour from our child. If we try to explain to her, she gets wild and rejects us. When I explain to her that something is not good for her, she is immediately supported by her grandparents who say that your mother doesn't know anything, you can do as you please. My daughter takes advantage of this and is now totally against me. She finds it easier to lead a life where nobody forces her to eat or study. I cannot quit working. How should I handle the situation? If I talk to my in-laws, they say they cannot take care of my daughter.

A. You do have a problem. But if you view it from a distance, you will see that your child is lucky to have caring parents and caring grandparents to look after her. In all families, there are some differences in the views of the two generations. Generally, the grandparents are considered to be over-indulgent by the parents of the child. The grandparents, on the other hand, feel that the parents are being unduly strict. You are in a situation that is common to many families.

However, it is only by changing your attitude slightly and by seeing the positive aspect of it can you begin to handle the situation. When you pick up your daughter in the evening, talk to her and let her talk to you. Do not use the time to instruct her on good behaviour and tell her what she ought to be doing. At age 4, there cannot be much studying to do. The time is meant for playing. Get her books and toys from which she can learn with enjoyment. Also if she is healthy, has the expected weight, and is active, there is no reason for you to be too worried about her eating. Of course, there is a problem if she has cold drinks all the time. Persuade her gently, when you have her on your lap and she is sure of your care and affection. Read stories to her, sing with her and play with her. If you constantly spend the little time you have in improving her, she will only become more adamant. Do everything gently and firmly. This will need patience. Try and find something good to say to your parents-in-law about their caring for the child, so that they treat the babysitting as a privilege, not a duty. Get your husband's cooperation in all the matters and give him some time or activity with the child, which is especially theirs. All the best.

49. How should I answer my son's questions regarding his father?

Q. I am a single working mother. My son is 5 years old and studying in class I. He does not know anything about his father as we separated before he was born. I live with my parents and brother and although my son is very happy, he feels the absence of his father and asks me questions about him. How do I tackle this? I do not want this problem to affect his studies or his life. Please advise.

A. It is unfortunate that you have not told anything about his father to your son or given him an opportunity to meet him. It is necessary to give an unbiased objective information to your son. Take care that you do not show the father in a poor light as it may affect your son's self-esteem. You can say that he loves you but due to some circumstances all fathers cannot live with the family. It is good that your son has an uncle and a grandfather around to provide male role models. But I feel that you should not deprive him of information about his father.

Sometimes children feel guilty and depressed for no fault of theirs. But in general, children are also much smarter and more tolerant than we think they are. It may be best to tell him the truth gently, at a suitable time, or you would spend much effort in covering one lie. Mother–child relationships are best built on a solid foundation of trust and confidence and this trust can carry over into future relationships as well. So do re-think your stand and reveal the truth gradually or at a suitable moment, assuring your son of your love.

50. Why is my 5-year-old not toilet trained as yet?

Q. **Recently, I caught my 5-year-old using the bathroom floor. He defecated on the bathroom floor and was urinating on his bedroom floor. When I confronted him he had no explanation for his behaviour. What could be causing him to do this?**

A. I think it is a serious problem and not related to the child's being toilet-trained. There are several points to be considered in handling this problem of your 5-year-old son defecating and urinating on the floor.

First, he may not be aware of the reason why he has done it. It reflects a serious psychological problem. He must be seen by an expert, as soon as possible. Please try to analyse the correlates of this incident. Is he suddenly afraid of something? Is he angry or resentful of an episode in the family? Sometimes children do such things simply to attract attention or to invite punishment. It is a signal of oppositional defiance.

Wait and watch, and maybe it might not get repeated. Tell him in simple words that it is undesirable behaviour. Do not ridicule him or beat him for it. Take his help in cleaning up. Above all, give him signals that you love him, but do not approve of this behaviour.

Do get him examined medically to rule out any physiological problem.

51. How can I raise my children properly as a single parent?

Q. **I am a single parent of two children aged 5 and 7 years. Their mother expired recently, last month. My children are very sensitive and shy. They are not so good in studies also. I am really worried about them. I am working in a private company and spend most of the time in office. My parents take care of them in my absence. There is a communication gap between my children and me. How can I take care of them and help them improve their self-confidence? Please advise something about their diet as well.**

A. Life can be quite tragic. But you must make sure that you spend enough time with the children, so that they know that you are there for them. Play with them and make them laugh. They should have plenty of toys to play with and books to read.

Food should be made palatable. Avoid spices, especially chillies. They should eat at least 4–5 times a day. Their preferences can be taken into account. They should not be forced to eat something, but persuaded to eat everything gradually. Talk to your parents and ask them how you can share in the rearing of the children. See if you can locate or set up a children's playgroup in your area, where all can meet on a Sunday afternoon. You could then discuss your doubts informally with other parents.

52. Does working of both parents affect the child's upbringing?

Q. I am a working woman with a 3-year-old son. My husband stays in Pune and comes home for weekends. We have a nuclear family. I have a full-time caretaker for my child. I need your guidance to learn about the parenting of my child. Does the non-availability of the father and mother affect emotional and mental growth of the child? Does the child feel rejected and can he blame the parents for not being available? What is the psychology of the child at this age? I feel guilty on these grounds. Am I wrong and what should I do?

A. Everything a child experiences is important for his full development. If the caretaker makes sure that the child has proper nourishing food, made and served attractively, his physical development will be all right. The child's intelligence is growing all the time. The more interesting and suitable his playthings are, the quicker his mind will develop. Speaking comes naturally to all children. They will repeat what they hear. They learn to speak the language spoken by others around them. There should be plenty of activities for your child's language to develop naturally. His relationship with you and his father is also very important and you must make sure that you spend as much time as you can spare, to talk to him, tell him stories, sing to him, feed him and play with him.

It is useless to feel guilty. It would be better to work for shorter hours in order to spend more time with your child, if you have the choice. Children want the mother and father more than anything. But this is a decision that you will have to make after you take note of all the factors and discuss the matter with your husband. If both of you can get jobs in the same city, some of the stress will be relieved.

Much depends on the caretaker you have appointed. If she is caring, affectionate, consistent and communicates well with the child, it is sheer good luck. I trust that you have trained her in meal preparation and the rules of hygiene. I hope that you are letting her go on leave during the weekends and doing the child's caregiving tasks yourself. That would ensure that the child develops attachment to you and associates you with fun and play as well.

53. What should I do to discipline my child?

Q. **My daughter is 4-and-a-half years old and is always playful, good at her studies, and gives no problem as such. As parents we are not able to make her lead a normal disciplined life. For example, even during night she continues playing. She does not like to go to the toilet regularly. Because of this she is always having health-related problems such as cold and constipation. Kindly advise.**

A. I am glad that your daughter is bright and playful. She is bound to have a good future. Playing is natural to children and it is the way they learn about things around them. However, you should be able to get a fairly simple routine going: fix specific times for meals and bedtime. You could make bedtime more interesting for her by reading stories to her or telling her stories. If you make that a routine, she will start looking forward to it and finish off other tasks first. Be gentle and firm with her, suggesting that you will give her more time, if she follows the basic rules.

Children sometimes get colds from drinking iced water or iced soft drinks. Encourage the child to eat fruits and vegetables and reduce the intake of biscuits etc. But since I don't know the child's weight, I should not suggest cutting out any item. I would rather suggest that you give her food that is well made, not too spicy, and full of vitamins. The child may not like to use the toilet because she is constipated; not vice versa. She might be hurting.

54. Our child is scared of us because we fight in front of him. What should we do?

Q. **My wife and I often fight in front of our 3-year-old son. He feels very insecure and is sometimes afraid to come near us. He cries a lot and is always sucking his fingers or thumb. I find all signs of depression in my wife. This usually is the reason for the quarrel. Sometimes, she becomes very violent. I am very tense about this. What will happen if it continues like this? What remedies should be taken to make my child normal?**

A. You should take help immediately not just for your wife and son, but also for the family interaction. Locate a good family therapist in your area or any psychiatrist or psychologist for a proper consultation. Meanwhile, avoid fighting in front of the child and have patience with your wife. A child can feel insecure and fearful, or may emulate aggressive behaviour if exposed to it often.

55. Why does my stepdaughter hate her mother?

Q. My stepdaughter is 3 years old. Her father and mother are going through a divorce right now. In the beginning, everyone had kept the baby out of it and now her mother has involved her. About 5 weeks ago, her mother took her from us for no reason and we didn't get to see her for 3 weeks. We did get to talk to her and she always wanted to come home to us. Her mother is very upset about it and has told her that she could not see or talk to us again. The baby is very angry with her. Well, we just got her back and she has not seen her mother in 2 weeks. We have tried getting her to talk to her on the phone but she refuses. She has even made comments like she hates her mother and doesn't like her and doesn't want to see her. We are very upset by this and don't know what to do. We don't talk about the divorce in front of the baby at all, and we definitely have not taught her to say it. So, my question is why is she saying these things? Why does she not want anything to do with her mother? Ever since we got her back she has been terrified of us leaving her alone; she throws a huge fit about it. We feel that she gets upset when we have to leave her with a babysitter because she is afraid that we won't come and get her.

A. The child is definitely insecure and perhaps suffering from attachment disruption. When the parents are going through divorce, the pain, anger and stress are likely to get displaced on to the child. The best option for you would be not to make the child self-conscious. Do not label the child as insecure. Your relaxed attitude will pass on a sense of security to her. Talk to her, play with her and hold her to comfort her. Do not force the child to go to the mother if she does not want to. Consult a child psychologist for help in dealing with the situation, if the problem persists.

56. How can I prevent my child from lying?

Q. How to stop my 3-year-old from lying?

A. It is important to find out why the child chooses not to speak the truth. If he is likely to be punished for the truth (e.g. he ate two of the biscuits after being told he cannot have them), it may be a matter of protecting himself. In this case, you should ensure that the punishment for his 'bad behaviour' is reasonable and not too strict. If he says he travelled in his friend's helicopter, it would be an instance of wishful thinking. Fantasy and reality can be easily mixed at this age. Observe what he says and does and do not be so quick to label everything as 'lying'.

However, there are some simple guidelines for preventing your child from lying:

- Serve as good role models yourself by speaking the truth in a non-hurting way.
- Encourage the child to speak the truth by rewarding desirable behaviour by praise or a hug.
- Tell stories depicting the advantages of being truthful and the drawbacks of lying. (*See also* page 61)

Speech disorders

57. Will my child always stammer?

Q. My daughter (3 years) has developed stuttering since the past 2 weeks and takes a lot of time to start a word or a sentence. She has absolutely no problems when she sings. She stammers on words like 'what' as wha-wha-what. Can you please guide us regarding the best approach to treat this problem? We have read extensively on this subject and we do not pressurize the child or correct her in between now. We let her talk and try to be calm when she stammers. As a background, since the past 2 months we tried to correct her words and tried to teach on how to hit the words or pronounce them so that her speech was clear. This I guess was the eagerness of parents. Our daughter is our first child and we are expecting our second baby in 3 months, which our daughter is aware of and we have been explaining her that she will soon have a baby sister/brother. Would this have caused stammering?

A. You seem to be very aware and well-read parents. The most important thing you can do to help your child is to be relaxed yourselves. Do not make her conscious of her mistakes, either through verbal or non-verbal reactions. Be good role models yourselves. Most children go through such phases and hopefully she will overcome it soon. Prepare her for the arrival of the new baby, but remember to continue attending to her needs too. Since the problem is only of the past 2 weeks, one can assume that it was triggered off by the emotional reaction to the news of the arrival of an addition to the family. However, if her speech continues to be less than normal, you might consult a speech therapist. (*See also* pages 57, 174)

Sex education

58. Why does my son keep questioning about private parts?

Q. My son is 5 years old. He doesn't feel shy in roaming without his briefs at home. I have tried telling him several times that it doesn't look nice and is not right. But nothing makes any difference to him. He still takes my help in wearing his clothes. One day he asked me pointing towards my breast that are you a fat lady and I said no, as I am average in weight and height. He then asked me that why do you and dadi have this? Why do papa and dadu don't have it? I replied that boys and girls are different. What should be my reply to him?

A. Young children do not feel shame regarding their physical features, and they are naturally as curious about private parts of the body, which are generally covered. With parental instruction and guidance, they gradually acquire social and cultural norms. They also observe people around them and imbibe acceptable conventions of behaviour. Their questions provide a good opportunity for parents to tell them about the facts of life at a level and in a language that they can understand.

Instead of feeling embarrassed about your child's questioning and instilling a sense of shame or guilt about his private parts, you can show him pictures and tell him how males and females are different. Household pets or farm animals often serve as examples for children to note sexual differences. You can tell him gently that some parts of the body have to be kept covered. You can also gradually warn the child about undesirable touch. If you give reasonable answers now, your child will trust you and will definitely turn to you in the future for resolving further doubts regarding sex and other issues. (*See also* page 50)

59. How can I stop my child from touching other people's breasts?

Q. My 4-year-old son has developed the habit of touching breasts of older people irrespective of their gender. He does this in a mischievous tone by verbally declaring his action. This behaviour followed after I stopped breastfeeding him at the age of one-and-a-half years. Earlier, this problem was not so severe, but of late, it has become very irritating. He does this mainly to the people in the house or to our close relatives when we visit them. But he doesn't exhibit this behaviour when unknown guests visit us. We have tried to make him understand that this type of behaviour is not good. We have also tried beating him for this, but there is no change in his behaviour. Please advise.

A. Your child's behaviour seems to be an attention-getting device. Instead of punishing him, use behaviour modification techniques.

First of all, try to ignore the undesirable behaviour. Instead give attention only to desirable actions. The child will quickly learn that some behaviour is not noticed and, therefore, useless.

Make a behaviour chart with him, where small lists of desirable and undesirable behaviour are clearly written. For every episode of breast touching etc., he gets a negative mark, while for every desirable behaviour he gets a red star. Red stars can be exchanged with a small gift at the end of the week.

Avoid labelling him as bad or dirty. Highlight his positive traits to encourage him. You can also tell him directly that his tendency to touch people's breasts is not acceptable. If he persists, his friends and relatives and so on will shun him. Hopefully you will gradually see a change in him.

Miscellaneous

60. Why does my daughter dislike to be called a girl?

Q. My daughter is 3-and-a-half years old. She is quite intelligent, mature and smart. The problem with her is that she does not like to identify herself as a girl, so much so that she does not want to wear a frock or similar dresses. She does not want us to introduce her as our daughter or even praise her as a 'good girl' or with similar words that categorize her as a girl. My mother-in-law stays with us. My daughter keeps saying that there are 2 female and 2 male members in our family. She counts herself as a male member. Our family is quite progressive and there is no gender bias at all. We are quite surprised with such an attitude. One thing that would be worth mentioning here is that she is very attached to her father and sometimes even asks how come her father is a boy and she a girl? Should we do something or just ignore her behaviour?

A. Children go through phases of gender-role identity adoption. It would be best to avoid arguing with her over gender issues. It is evident that she is identifying with her father and, therefore, wants to think of herself as a boy. She is declaring this identification, and perhaps showing rebellious attitude. As she grows older, you can expect a change. Peer pressure and identification with same-sex parent would occur on its own. Meanwhile, since you do not have gender bias, it may be possible to refrain from expecting 'girlish' behaviour for some time and not referring to her as a girl. Try not to make it a power issue or take it as a personal insult. Exposure to appropriate gender stereotypes, family discussion and debate over gender issues when she is older, and her own need for peer conformity would gradually prove useful in helping her accept herself.

61. How should I deal with my daughter getting upset about my going to work?

Q. **My 4-year-old daughter has these phases when she is extremely upset about my going to work. She behaves in an extremely aggressive way with everyone at home and becomes unmanageable at times. The mood lasts for about a week and then she gets over it. But this is repeated after a couple of weeks. Earlier, I could relate this behaviour to the periods when I spent more hours at work. But she goes through these separation pangs even though I have stopped working late hours and now ensure that I give adequate attention to her everyday. What is the best way to handle these situations and to create a positive thinking in her mind about my going to work?**

A. The memory of missing you is still vivid in your child's mind, even though you are more available to her. But since her tantrums had the effect she had hoped for, she may think that a little more show of temper on her part might bring you back for longer hours. When you are with her, give her close attention, talk to her. Tell her that you love her, but you also have to be away at work. Let her talk to you. While you are cooking, for example, she can be in the same room with a cup and spoon, making up a game. Use that time to listen to her. Everything is gradual. She will settle down to the changed routine after a while.

A lot also depends on the arrangements you have made for her when you are not there. If you leave her with a domestic worker or paid caregiver, please ensure that the situation is comfortable for your child and that she is well looked after. In life, there are no formula solutions. Most of these problems require affection, patience and firmness on the part of parents. (*See also* page 92)

62. How can I make my daughter adjust to the fact of being the only child?

Q. **My daughter is 5 years old. She has lately started imagining having a little brother or sister to play with. Most of her friends have had a baby being born in their house. Now, she is telling people that I am pregnant and she and the baby will sleep in one room. She says that she has prayed to God and it will definitely come true, even though I have told her the opposite. I am almost 40 years old and have no plans for another child. How do I deal with her needs? Do single children grow up to be lonely or have other emotional problems? Presently, she seems to be well adjusted and happy, though**

slightly shy and timid. What can I do to make up for the fun she misses out on growing up with siblings? I get her to socialize as much as possible. How can I help her adjust to the reality that she's a single child?

A. Many children have imaginary playmates when they are lonely. What your little girl is doing is expressing what she would wish, as if it were a fact. You could arrange for her to have her age mates in the neighbourhood or classmates come and play with her. If there are cousins, they could also be interacting with her more frequently, so that it becomes like a sibling bond. All these would not be a substitute for a real baby in the house; but she will have to accept the reality. There are many people who have grown up well and happy as being the only child. Being an only child is not a problem in itself.

Some parents consider adoption of a child to provide a companion for their child, but such a decision has to be taken after proper deliberation and discussion.

Guide her to an interesting extracurricular activity, where she can meet other children in a reasonably informal setting (art class, playgroup, music class, etc.). Your child has a vivid imagination. You could make puppets and let her tell stories to other children. You will have to work out some activity that she enjoys doing and where her talents find an expression. (*See also* page 93)

63. Is my child exhibiting inappropriate behaviour or is it just play?

Q. I have a 3-year-old son. Most of his milestones were late. He started walking after 2 years and now he speaks 2–3 words at a time but not as well as other children of his age. As both my husband and I are working, he stays with my mother during the day. He is going to the nursery class. Last week, his teacher complained about him and said that he is very fond of a particular girl in the class and keeps hugging and kissing her. She has observed this for some weeks now. She says he sits on the girl and plays with her. The teacher says he must have seen something of this kind on the TV. She says I should speak to him and ask him where and how he has seen this or why he is doing this. But I can't ask him anything of this kind since he is too small to answer or understand my questions? I don't see anything wrong in his attitude. When we come home after work, he hugs us, kisses us and even if we lie down, he will sit on us and play with us. We have tried to restrict him from doing this but it is a kind of play for him. I don't know how to tackle

this problem. Should I go to a child psychologist or a speech therapist?

A. Since your child has a delay in developmental milestones, it is quite likely that he does not understand how his playful actions can be interpreted. But you will agree that the little girl's parents can be a little disturbed if a boy in her class is too friendly with her.

Perhaps you should discourage your son from playing certain kinds of games with you, such as sitting on you when you are prone. What is appropriate when a child is 1 or even 2 begins to look odd in a child of 3 years of age. Get him a big soft ball that he can play with. Join him in the game when you can. Put on music and let him move (dance) to the tunes. Spend time teaching him to use words for his actions. Indicate what is good and what is not. Children will absorb parental rules in everyday activities. They want the approval of parents and teachers. Children start speaking as they grow up. Speech develops rapidly when the child encounters people and playthings and needs to communicate.

Suggest to the teacher in the nursery school that she should distract him and present other things to do, when the child starts to dominate (or even monopolize) the selected friend in the school. He has to be clearly told what the boundaries are for his freedom. This must be done gently but firmly and parents are the best adults to do this.

If you have access to a psychologist who specializes in children's problems, you might wish to consult her. If your home remedies (or acting on my suggestions) do not work, that is of course an option. In the meantime, start interesting games and plenty of activities for the child at home, while the parents are away at work.

64. How can one handle a child's crying when her mother leaves for work?

Q. My friend is separated and lives with her parents who attend to her 4-year-old daughter. She is a working woman and of late her daughter cries profusely and throws a tantrum when she leaves for work. What is the best way to handle this situation?

A. Since you say that of late the little girl has started crying when her mother leaves for work, you must try and find out what circumstance has changed recently. Did the child start attending (or change) a preschool or playcentre? Did the family sack an old 'ayah' and get a new one? With no background facts of any kind to help me, I am unable to offer any suggestion.

Maybe the mother should take off a couple of days and see what activities her daughter is involved in and who her companions/friends are. Also, a 4-year-old has fully developed language and she can be asked why she is distressed. This should not be done at the time she is upset, but when she is relaxed and playing.

Crying is the language children use when they are upset. The best way of handling the situation is to locate the cause of distress. If the mother has to go out to work, it is part of reality that the child will ultimately accept. Patience and time are essential. (*See also* page 90)

65. Is it normal for a child to have an invisible friend?

Q. My 5-year-old grandson has had an invisible buddy for several months. Here is an example of a situation that happened today. There was no power in the house last night due to a snake that got into a substation. When my grandson learnt this, he started crying and said it was his invisible buddy's pet who is dead. He had acted up at school today and when asked what was bothering him he looked at his buddy and looked back at his mom and said 'Because a puny snail is in my brain'. When asked how to get it out. He looked at his buddy and back at his mom and said by doing a wet willy (a wet willy is where you stick your finger in your mouth and get it wet then stick in your ear). His mom asked if she needed to give him a wet willy and he said no he could do it himself. So, he gave himself a wet willy. His mom asked if he got it and he looked at his buddy and asked if he could have the puny magnifying glass. He took it from his buddy and pretending to hold an object, he was looking at his finger. He said he got it unless he had two. Is this normal for a child to have an invisible buddy?

A. It is perfectly normal for a 5-year-old to have an imaginary playmate. As the child grows up, he will outgrow the idea. There is no cause for worry about an imaginary buddy. Probably, the books and stories read out to the child have a great deal of fantasy and it is normal for children to create characters that they wish could be real. One could call it wishful thinking.

He may be missing siblings or other children to play with. Perhaps you should look into the possibility of introducing joint playing sessions with your grandson and one or two children in the neighbourhood after school hours. In any case, one should not make an issue of the child having an imaginary playmate. You can play along a bit, but also bring in real-life interesting events for the child. Introduce a variety of activities, so that choices can be made by the child according to his inclination and taste.

You should be glad that the child has such a rich imagination. As he grows up, he can really go places!

66. Why does my son get very excited when guests come?

Q. My son is nearly 3-and-a-half years old. He cries a lot during evening and speaks a lot at nights. He always wants to watch the POGO channel and it is impossible for us to watch another channel. I have also noticed that in the absence of his father, he never asks for him at all. Is this normal? When I beat him sometimes, he says that he'll complain to his father. He started speaking very late but can speak 2 languages now. He hates studying, but otherwise he is a very affectionate and normal. Do children normally get excited when a guest comes home? He loves playing with other children of his age. He has a wheezing problem and refuses to take ice cream or chocolate and says, 'Mummy, I will get a cold'. Is this quite normal?

A. Children are sensitive to family interactions. Is the father absent for long periods? Has there been bonding between the father and son? Are there arguments or conflicts between you and your husband, especially in the evenings, which make him feel insecure? Speaking a lot at night could be due to anxiety or bad dreams.

It is normal to be happy and excited when guests come. Guests may be a signal for him that he will not be forced or scolded while they are there, so he may feel relieved and happy. It is also normal to want to play. On the other hand, it is not normal to expect a 3-year-old to 'study'. He seems to be an intelligent child who is careful about what he eats so that he doesn't fall ill. You are lucky that he knows what is not good for him; most parents have the reverse problem of keeping away unsuitable food items.

From the details provided by you, it seems that you are rather assertive and tend to force him to do what you want. Perhaps you were critical of him when he started speaking late. It is entirely unnecessary to beat him. Gentle persuasion will be more effective. Beating him or forcing him to study or watch a certain channel will only lead to resentment. Fix a time limit for his watching TV. POGO is certainly more appropriate for his age than adult programmes. Try and get him to bed as early as possible, by about 8 p.m. Reduce the noise level in the home and let him sleep early.

He would be happy to have affectionate, firm and consistent parenting. Reward him for his positive efforts and provide a calm, loving and secure environment at home.

67. What should I do to protect my son from child abuse?

Q. **What could be the cause of lip licking? Whenever my son comes back from a weekend visit to his father, he has a severely chapped area around his mouth, which is red, scaly and raw. I treat it with Vaseline as per the paediatrician's suggestion, yet it reappears after the next visit. Someone told me this could be a sign of abuse. My son is very anxious about the time spent with his father. He complains of stress during mealtimes, such as being forced to eat food he doesn't like, in large quantities so that he vomits; not being allowed to go to the bathroom when he needs to go; no heating in the house in cold months and sleeping on the floor in his father's room with the television going on all night. Are all these signs of child abuse?**

A. What you say sounds very much like child abuse. Please do not send your child to the father. You may need to get the help of a lawyer and if possible some organization for the protection of children, such as the Indian Council for Child Welfare. There is a telephone helpline that you can access, if your child is being abused. Also speak to the elders in the family and neighbours, who will support you in your decision not to let the child visit the father and experience such abuse. If you are hesitant to go to a lawyer, try legal aid.

In any case, do not keep this matter to yourself; share it with others. Many problems get solved when they are exposed to the public. Do not suffer in silence, but take courage and expose the matter after you have taken precautions to protect yourself and the child. What the child's father is doing is horrible and unforgivable. I guess that it must be his way of punishing you for asking for a separation/divorce. I do not know where you live or what your resources are, so my advice cannot be more specific. Surely there must be someone you can reach out to at this time, to keep your son from being abused. Think about everything coolly, with deliberation and then take action. Remember, an abusive father, who literally tortures his young son must be denied visiting rights. Get your child out of being regularly at the receiving end of such gruesome experiences.

68. Why does my child speak to herself but is unable to express to others?

Q. My question relates to my daughter who is 5 years old. As per my observation and from the feedback from school, she is intelligent and selectively active, i.e. she is active in certain environments. But of late, I have been noticing in her some of the traits which I carried in my childhood, particularly, speaking to oneself even in public places like malls. Is this a habit to be curtailed or should I ignore it. Your guidance on this topic will be highly appreciated. Secondly, during the PTA meeting a passing comment was made by the teacher regarding her inability to express her thoughts in spite of her knowing the subject. I noticed the same much earlier. She feels free to express her thoughts only to me. Is there a way to overcome this?

A. Children at age 5 are still in the process of developing their vocabulary and grammatical skills. This makes them inhibited sometimes. They differ in inhibition levels and are often able to express themselves better to a parent. Your daughter is too young for you to worry about the issue. Instead of making her conscious about it, try to encourage her when she reports that she said something in the class. Do not criticize her, as it would make her more inhibited.

Regarding the habit of speaking to herself, this is another characteristic of children at this age. Children find it easier to verbalize their thoughts rather than thinking in an abstract way. Since you remember you had the same habit, but have emerged as a normal person, perhaps there is no reason to worry about it. If the habit persists or increases, maybe you can get her assessed by a child psychologist.

69. How can I help my daughter get rid of her fear?

Q. My 5-year-old daughter always remains scared. When she was 1 year old, she used to cry when she saw someone in a black dress. She did not mingle much with other people and preferred to play alone. She overcame this but is still reserved. She is still scared of things. She does not play in the swimming pool. If we go out, she does not like rain. I explained her things when she saw about the tusnami on TV. If we talk about death or she sees an accident on TV, she gets scared. I avoid letting her watch TV and talk about such matters. Last week she saw an accident on TV. She keeps questioning me whether all people are nice? Do accidents take place everywhere? I am a working woman and my parents look after her. My husband and I make it a point to

spend much time with her. I have stopped watching TV or movies. I ask her questions about what she did in school, how are her friends. I am a little disciplined. I point out wrong things and ask her to correct them. She is good in academics and her teacher always says good things about her. They recently told me that her confidence has increased tremendously from the time she started going to school. Her doctor says she is perfectly fine. Should I go for counselling?

A. Your own behaviour seems contradictory. On the one hand, you try to explain about tsunami or death to her, and on the other hand you have stopped watching TV with her. The security and confidence level of a child is determined by the stability of attachment with the mother and father. Maybe your child would benefit from a higher sense of security. This can be achieved through closer bonding and spending time with her. Many children of her age are afraid of trying out new things. As a parent, you cannot protect your child forever from the realities of the outside world. Instead, you should try and make her stronger to enable her to face the harsh realities well.

It seems that her school environment has a good stabilizing influence on her emotions. She will hopefully overcome her fears. In case she does not improve, you can consult a counsellor or child psychologist. (*See also* page 44)

70. My granddaughter strangled her pet bird, what should we do?

Q. Our daughter dropped our 4-year-old granddaughter saying she could not take her home. Our daughter raises doves. Four days ago they got a Minx kitten. Our granddaughter strangled the kitten 2 days ago. Our daughter also told us that the child had strangled a baby dove a week and a half ago. I asked the child why she did it, and she replied that it was just sitting there. I asked her if she realized her mistake and she said that she did. We have 3 miniature dachshunds and I caught her with her hands around a dog's throat. I asked her what she was doing and she said that she was just patting the dog. But I don't think so. What should we do with this child?

A. From a simple reading of the situation, I think the 4-year-old girl feels something similar to sibling rivalry for all the little animals being brought up in the two homes. It seems to me that the child is craving for the attention of her mother and grandmother and finds that the animals are in the way. Her hatred for the animals will not fall in the category of cruelty to animals.

You may have to find ways of engaging the little girl in activities of her choice and also assure her that you do love her. Under the circumstances, provision for daycare, where there are other children of her age, may be a good alternative. Do talk to a psychologist or counsellor, if you think you need to, for further advice, but do not treat the child as a killer of animals. She needs to play with toys and have stories read to her. If you could put her happiness on priority, the problem may get solved.

71. Why is my child obsessed with one kind of play?

Q. I am 32 years old and have one son who is 4-and-a-half years old. He is going to school for the past one year. My concern is that my son always tries to play with a bow and arrow. I tried to find out the problem. I figured out that when he was younger my wife always use to say 'you will become strong like Lord Ram'. Please suggest me how I can handle this problem? He always tries to mould paper, copy, pencil, etc. in the form of an arrow or bow.

A. Children go through phases of interests, and explore identities. Why are you upset with his preoccupation with bows and arrows or wanting to become like Lord Ram? If you get more upset with such behaviour, the situation is likely to turn into a power struggle. Many children make arrows out of paper and watch them flying! You could also try and provide other play materials, which the child can use. You should try to ignore the behaviour which is annoying and try to distract his attention. But wanting to be strong and God-like is hardly anything one should worry about. Do not scold or criticize him unnecessarily. On the other hand, reward him by a smile, hug or verbal encouragement when he finds new ways to amuse himself. And don't forget that he is only 4 years old.

6 to 9 year olds

- Disciplining children
- Safety tips
- Sexual abuse
- The child at school

- School issues
- Disciplining children
- Sex education
- Fears

Disciplining children

How do you discipline a child of this age?

Ages 0 to 2

Babies and toddlers are naturally curious, and the best way to discipline a young child is to eliminate temptations. A child who has been hitting, biting, or throwing food, should be told why that behaviour is unacceptable. Try to calm him for a minute or two.

Never spank, hit or slap a child of any age. Babies and toddlers are especially unlikely to be able to make any connection between their behaviour and the physical punishment. They will only feel the pain. Do not forget that children learn by watching you. Make sure that your behaviour is perfect as it has a strong impact on the child's behaviour.

Ages 3 to 5

As your child grows, he begins to understand the connection between actions and consequences. It is important to explain to him what you expect of him before you punish him for a certain behaviour. For instance, the first time your child uses crayons to decorate the living room wall, you should discuss why that is not allowed and what will happen if it's done again. Explain to him that he will have to help keep the walls clean. If he repeats this act again, you should remind him that crayons are for paper only and then enforce the consequences.

It is easier for parents to ignore bad behaviour occasionally. But, it is important for you as parents to decide together what the rules are and then be consistent in upholding them. There should be clarity on what behaviour will be punished; do not forget to reward good behaviour. Discipline is not just about punishment. Parents need to remember to recognize and reward good behaviour as well.

Ages 6 to 8

Timeouts and consequences are effective discipline strategies with this age group. Consistency is important at this stage. The child should be made to believe that you mean what you say.

You should try and follow through with what you say. Be careful not to make unrealistic threats of punishment in anger, since not following through will put you in the difficult position of not being able to carry out your threat. Severe punishments may be counter-productive. The child may not feel motivated to change his behaviour.

Ages 9 to 12

The child in this age group, just as with all ages, can be disciplined with natural consequences. As he matures and requests for more independence and responsibility, teaching him to deal with the consequences of his behaviour is an effective and appropriate disciplining technique. For example, if your child has not done his homework before bedtime and goes to school without it the next day, he faces the consequences. He will realize automatically what behaving improperly can mean, and will probably not make those mistakes again. However, if your child does not seem to be learning from natural consequences, you should set up your own consequences to help him modify his behaviour more effectively.

Ages 13 and above

By now your child knows what is expected of him and knows that you mean what you say about the consequences of bad behaviour. Don't let down your guard now, as discipline is just as important for teens as it is for younger children. Make sure to set up rules regarding homework, visits by friends, and discuss them beforehand with your teenager so that there will be no misunderstandings. He will probably complain from time to time, even as you grant him greater freedom and responsibility.

When your child does break a rule, taking away privileges may seem to be the best plan of action. It is also important to give a teenager some control over his life. It will help him to respect the decisions you make for him.

What is positive discipline?

The key to success is for parents to establish their authority over the child without putting them on the offensive and getting into a power struggle. Children, just like other people, do not react well to taking orders. The instinct is to rebel and the parents' automatic reaction is to exert further pressure. The child must get the message that discipline is for his own good.

Many a time, children distract their parents with their naughtiness and disobedience. On such occasions, parents may see no other option but to give the children a good spanking. While this does not cause serious damage if it is a rare occurrence, it has been observed that children whose parents discipline them by hitting, nagging or shouting at them on a regular basis, have a tendency to be more violent and aggressive than other children who are disciplined through other means.

Another important thing that parents should keep in mind is that when they rebuke their child, they should make them understand that it is a specific behaviour that is under criticism and not the child himself. The child must feel that he is not a bad person, but that he has not behaved correctly in a particular situation.

Punishment should be aimed at making children understand the consequences of their actions and to take responsibility for their actions.

How to deal with a stubborn child?

Stubbornness in children has always been viewed as a negative trait by parents. But maybe they should attempt to look upon it in a more positive fashion. A child's stubbornness may just be his way of demonstrating that he can think for himself. Stubbornness gives him a feeling that he has a measure of control over the situation, which in turn, boosts his self-esteem. Parents should also make an effort to understand the root of their children's stubbornness. Stubbornness can have a range of causes. It may vary from irrational fears to resistance to change or just a simple attack of rebellion. Do not get angry or argue with them. Simply state your stand, the reasons for it and the consequences of disobedience. Then follow through. If the issue is not serious, there is no harm negotiating with your child and arriving at a compromise. In some situations, it may be more effective to just let go without any opposition.

Some useful tips

- Identify the problem and involve your child in seeking a solution. In this way he will feel that you are on his side.
- If you want your child to do something, try to time your request so that it does not interrupt him while he is doing something else. This is one way of avoiding a conflict.
- If your child is not very happy about a change, give him adequate notice so that he knows what to expect and is willing to cooperate.
- Be assertive when asking your child to do something. You are not asking him for a favour. Also, make clear the consequences of non-compliance.
- Keep in mind that your requests should be reasonable. Praise your child when he is cooperative and well behaved.

Safety tips

Playing in the sun

Young children

- Babies under 6 months of age should be kept out of direct sunlight, i.e. in the shade.
- Dress babies in light clothing that covers the arms and legs.
- Apply sunscreen at least 30 minutes before going outside, and use sunscreen even on cloudy days.

Older children

The best defence against the sun is covering up. Wear a hat with a three-inch brim or a shade facing forward, sunglasses (look for sunglasses that block ultraviolet rays), and cotton clothing with a tight weave. Stay in the shade whenever possible, and avoid sun exposure during peak intensity hours (from 10 a.m. to 4 p.m.). The risk of sunburn increases at higher altitudes.

Sunscreen with an SPF (sun protection factor) of 15 should be effective for most people. Be sure to apply enough sunscreen. Reapply sunscreen every two hours, or after swimming or sweating. Creams or baby oil may make the skin look shiny and soft, but they provide no protection from the sun.

Swimming pool safety

- Never leave children alone in or near the pool.
- Make sure an adult trained in life-saving techniques is close at hand.
- Avoid inflatable swimming aids such as 'floaties'.
- Life vests can give children a false sense of security.

Bicycle safety

- Do not push your child to ride a 2-wheeled bicycle until he is ready, at about age 5 or 6. Consider the child's coordination and desire to learn to ride. Stay with support wheels on both sides until your child is older and more experienced.
- Take your child with you when you shop for the bike, so that he can try it out. The value of a properly sized bike far outweighs the value of surprising your child with a new bike.
- Buy a bike that is the right size, not one your child has to 'grow into'. Oversized bikes are especially dangerous.

Test the bicycle for proper fit

- Sitting on the seat with hands on the handlebar, your child must be able to place the balls of both feet on the ground.

- Straddling the centre bar, your child should be able to stand with both feet flat on the ground with about a 1-inch clearance between the crotch and the bar.
- When buying a bike with hand brakes for an older child, make sure that the child can comfortably grasp the brakes and apply sufficient pressure to stop the bike. A helmet should always be worn while riding bikes.

Sexual abuse

What is sexual abuse?

Sexual abuse in children is a term used when the offender, who may or may not be a member of the family, uses a child for his sexual gratification. Very young children as well as older teenagers may be victimized.

What does sexual abuse include?

Sexual abuse can be physical, verbal or emotional and includes the following:

- Touching and fondling with sexual intent.
- Exposing children to adult sexual activity or pornographic material.
- Having children pose, undress or perform in a sexual fashion on film or in person.
- 'Peeping' into bathrooms or bedrooms to spy on a child.
- Rape or attempted rape.

The perpetrator may use force, tricks, bribes or threats to involve a child into sexual activity. The use of physical force however is rarely necessary because children wish to seek love and approval from adults, and believe that adults are always right.

What are the signs of sexual abuse?

Children generally do not tell if they are being sexually abused because they may be afraid of the perpetrator. The abuser may threaten to harm the child or any member of her family if she told them. In cases, where the abuser is known to the child, he may ask her not to divulge 'their little secret' to anyone else.

Parents or guardians must be vigilant towards their children since there are certain general behaviour changes that may occur in children if they are experiencing such a problem.

- Sleep disturbances
- School problems
- Withdrawal from family, friends or usual activities
- Other problems may include depression, anxiety, discipline problems, drug or alcohol problems, hostility or aggression and in some cases running away.

Children who have been sexually abused frequently have more specific symptoms such as displaying sexual knowledge or behaviour that is beyond what is normal for their age; copying adult sexual behaviour;

unexplained pain, swelling, bleeding or irritation of the mouth; urinary infections and sexually transmitted infections.

How does a sexually abused child feel?

A sexually abused child may feel different emotions such as fear of the abuser or of being different from other children; anger at other adults around her who did not protect her; isolation, sadness, guilt, confusion and shame.

What should parents do?

As concerned adults, parents should teach the children:

- that they are loved, valued and are very precious.
- the difference between good and bad touches.
- that their bodies belong to them and nobody has the right to touch or hurt them.
- to tell their parents everything about which they feel uncomfortable.

If a child trusts her parents and tells them about the incident, they should help by providing positive support.

Some dos:

- Keep calm.
- Believe the child.
- Give positive messages such as 'I know you could not help it', 'I'm proud that you trusted me'.
- Respect the child's privacy and never discuss the topic in front of others.
- Take the child for a medical check-up to make sure that no permanent damage has occurred.

Some don'ts:

- Never panic or overreact as the child needs help and support through this difficult time.
- Never confront the offender in the child's presence.
- Do not blame the child because sexual abuse is never the child's fault.

The child at school

Many people think that school is a place where the child learns to read, write, do arithmetic, memorize facts about geography, history and science. It is, however, much more than this. A school is not just a place where the child learns these subjects. It is also a place where he learns to get on with people and is thus preparing for adult life. Going to school, for many children, is the first experience outside their home. The child begins to be part of a group outside his family. School forms a very important part in the character building of a child. Experiences in school are wide and varied. The child comes into contact with other children of different religions, beliefs and values.

Which school to choose?

When parents decide that the child is ready for regular school and they wish to choose one for him, they should not only look at the school's results but also the type of students the school has produced. It is also important to see the extent to which the school has helped prepare the children for their future.

For younger children, schools should preferably be in the same locality or neighbourhood. Long travel in school buses or city transport for an hour or more can tire and exhaust the child leading to apathy, headache and many other illnesses.

Different schools have different mediums for education. The medium of language is very important. A good student in an English medium school may find himself at a disadvantage if the medium is changed.

Parents sometimes debate about sending their children to a boarding school. There may be special reasons for this. It is important to note that in the early years, the child needs the warmth and security of being with his family. Beyond age 11 or 12, most children are independent and can look after themselves. Children who are difficult to manage at home or undisciplined are often sent to a boarding school. This is not correct as the child takes it as a punishment, and develops greater hostility or increased guilt feelings. The child may distance himself from the family and may have adjustment problems later.

When to put the child in school?

There is no harm in sending a 3-year-old to a nursery school in the neighbourhood where there are other children to play with, to talk with and to have fun. Such schools enable a child to be on his own and to face problems without the protection of parents. The nursery school is primarily meant for playing and learning to be social. If you feel that your child is happy playing at home and with children in the neighbourhood, it is not necessary to push him to school at an early stage. You can wait until he is 5 years old to put him in the kindergarten class or a regular school.

What are the problems that children face while going to school?
Some children feel nervous or even scared on the first day of school because of all the new things: new teachers, new friends, and maybe even a new school. When a child first starts going to school, he may feel reluctant or cry when you leave him at the school gates. Not every child is prepared to accept school at the same age. A lot depends on his experiences in playing with other children and meeting strange people. A child who plays with other children will not have much difficulty in going to a school, whereas a child who is always playing with his mother or does not have too many children to play with, will resent the idea of separation from the mother.

Normally, the first child usually has school problems. In such cases, where there is strong resentment, it is best not to push the child, otherwise he is likely to develop permanent aversion to school. Go with the child to the school for a couple of days and give him the reassurance that you will not disappear, but will meet him when the school finishes. Slowly, he will adjust to his new environment.

In an older child, the reluctance to go to school may be due to bullying or teasing at school. Sometimes it follows an illness or a prolonged absence from the school or punishment by the teacher. He may start having problems such as headache, pain in the abdomen or vomiting. Changing the school is not usually helpful in these cases. At times there can be excessive teasing at school that can cause unhappiness. Causes of teasing include inability to pronounce words correctly, social class, clumsiness and obesity. Some children who try to please the teacher are often teased for being the teacher's pet. Such children are usually overprotected at home and lack normal aggressive behaviour.

What is the role of parents?
A parent should be concerned, though not overprotective about her child. Take active interest in his school activities, in his examination results, and discuss school with him. Find out how he feels about being in school and who his friends are. Most schools have parent–teacher meeting once a term and parents must make it a point to attend such meetings. Many parents are ignorant about the class or section of their children. Most parents visualize the child at school from their own experience. This may not be the best way.

They should look at the school from the child's point of view, and how he relates to his surroundings and feels about the different issues.

What if the child is performing badly at school?
When your child is doing badly at school, do not blame the school or the teacher. There may be many reasons for it. He may have been put into school too early or he may be too young for his class and may have to compete with older children. The other reasons may be that he has missed many days at school because of illness in early childhood.

At times, home environment is responsible for the child's bad performance in school. Quarrelling parents, or a home where the child does not get enough love, or the birth of another child which takes away the attention of parents, can also be responsible for the child's poor performance. There is also the possibility that he may not be getting along well with his teacher. If you suspect this, have a talk with the principal and discuss the problem with him tactfully.

Some parents give the wrong age of the child to the school authorities in an attempt to push him to a higher class. This attitude is not healthy. If the child is a year or two younger than other children in the class, he may have difficulty in adjusting. A 4-year-old child will be less mature and have far less understanding than a 5-year-old. Similarly, a double promotion saves a year but taxes the child. A child doing well in one class may not be as good in the other class. This creates unnecessary resentment, pressure and a feeling of inadequacy in the child.

How to help the child cope with examinations?
These are the days of competition. The child has to succeed in many competitions and examinations. The importance of examinations has increased to such an extent that the years between 10–17 are spent in constant fear of them. Parents, instead of helping, invariably increase the fear psychosis in their children, resulting in serious personality problems.

Parents should reassure their children regarding examinations and not increase their anxiety. They should help the child in his schoolwork when he has any difficulty. Although you can help him with his homework, you cannot take the examinations for him. In the long run, it will only make things more difficult for him. You should help him when he cannot understand or comprehend something but do not make him over-dependant on you. He should be encouraged to do his homework regularly.

School issues

72. Is my child a slow learner?

Q. I started to realize that my only 8-year-old child might be a slow learner (I am not so sure of that yet). I have no problem in accepting this but my dilemma is how can I deal with it, if it is found so? His self-confidence is very low, he cries a lot and for all silly reasons. He is unable to cope with new situations and can't deal well with his friends. There are some kids in the neighbourhood of his age but he doesn't like to play with them. He is afraid and incapable of competing with kids of his age. As for school, he doesn't like to study and his handwriting looks like that of a 6-year-old. He skips letters while writing (in both Arabic and English), in addition to some difficulties in reading and in maths. Please note that I am a single parent, and I am tense most of the times. I end up yelling and get nervous. Your help will be highly appreciated.

A. It is not surprising that your child has some problems with reading and writing, since you made him learn two languages – English which goes from left to right and Arabic which goes from right to left. Errors in writing should not be taken so seriously.

At the outset, you must try to introspect if, as a single parent, you are being over-anxious and over-protective in dealing with your only child and unconsciously making him dependent on you. That may have reduced his confidence. Your being tense and yelling at him cannot improve the situation. If you express affection and tenderness and let him tell you what he feels, his self-confidence will improve. Do his teachers have the same opinion of him? In case a change is required in your own parenting style, you should make an attempt to do so. If he still does not show much improvement, it would be advisable to consult a child psychologist or counsellor.

73. How can I inculcate the habit of reading in my child?

Q. **My son is 7 years old. I want him to read books and to inculcate in him the habit of reading. He is not interested in reading. I have bought him several books but he does not seem to be interested. How can I inculcate the reading habit in my child?**

A. These days, children are moving away from reading due to several reasons. They have enough reading to do for school studies. Then there are many distractions such as television and computer, which leave no time or patience for reading.

To encourage good reading habits in your child, you should first of all serve as a good example yourself. If the child finds you reading instead of being glued to television, he may also want to do the same.

Providing appropriate reading material, controlling television viewing and helping the child to structure his routine to include enough time to play and read will help. Nagging a child to read is not desirable as it may make the child rebel. He will read only if he finds it interesting and valuable. Buy a lot of attractive story books for him and give him a chance to talk about what he read, at mealtimes or other family gatherings.

74. Why does my daughter stay aloof and refuse to go to school?

Q. **My daughter is 6 years old. She is an intelligent and affectionate girl but has migraine, which affects her routine. She is under medication (homoeopathy) for the past one year. Last year she had a bout of gastroenteritis after which she refused to go to school. She creates a big fuss over studies and homework. She is a poor eater and skips her lunch during school. She doesn't do anything on her own, unless somebody helps her. She lacks concentration and cribs and complains about everything. She doesn't like any kind of physical activity. She is glued to the TV all the time. She is afraid of staying alone even for 10 seconds. She questions a lot and keeps repeating it, though she knows the answer. She does not like to mingle with other children. She is becoming adamant. She loves playing on her own and talking to herself. She doesn't have siblings. Her teacher says**

that she disturbs (helps) others rather than doing her job. What should we do? I am worried about her behaviour.

A. Since many of your child's problems seem to be rooted in her health, it would be necessary to have a complete check-up of her physical system. Her more recent bout of gastroenteritis seems to have made her unwilling to go to school. Maybe the bathrooms in the school are not convenient, or the helpers in the school are unwilling to take her to the toilet when she wants to go. I think you should let her speak to you and listen to her carefully. Ask her what happened, indicating that you will help her. Do this gently over a period of time and not in an authoritarian style.

Children who do not have any siblings often have imaginary playmates. If she is helping others in her class, that is a nice trait. Instead of trying to change her into a normal child, maybe you could see what her nature is and where her interests lead and then try to work around them. Spend time with her in a way that is enjoyable for her and for you.

Try to avoid cola drinks for your child. In fact all aerated or soft drinks can be avoided. Coffee and tea should not be a part of her diet. Her TV watching should be selective and not more than an hour a day.

After the initial period of getting adjusted to the school, children like to attend school. You must find out why your daughter is not happy to go to school. The problem may not be of her making. Be patient and check out everything.

75. Will my son's interest in drawing affect his academics?

Q. My 6-year-old son has a keen interest in drawing and painting. Seeing his inclination, we arranged for him a drawing teacher. However, we find that he is more interested in drawing than his studies. He used to be a better student before. But his performance has deteriorated in academics. I thought of meeting his class teacher and wanted to request for an appointment via his school diary. But he told me not to do so. Even when I did write, he did not show it to his teacher. In the drawing classes, he doesn't take interest in the methodology followed by the drawing teacher but wants to draw cartoon characters etc. and scribbles them in his copy as per his choice. Will his deep interest in drawing divert his attention from academics? Is he trying to be independent in his decisions by not showing his diary to his teacher? He is generally well behaved but sometimes shows aggression. Is it normal for children of 10 years to do so? He is asthmatic and takes Beclate regularly along with homoeopathic medicines.

A. In the opening sentence, you say that your son is 6 years old. At the end of query, you make him 10 years old. I am not very clear, which is the right age.

If he is only 6 years old, you do not have to worry about academics. Even if he is 10, the school must be ensuring some coverage of the subjects. Children learn from every activity and there is no hierarchy of subjects. I think that a 6-year-old, who is good at drawing just needs encouragement. He needs large sheets of paper, colours, both crayons and paints, materials of different textures, which he can feel and make into collage or small objects. And plenty of chalk and smooth floors on which he can scribble. In my experience, drawing teachers may teach a child some technique, but they tend to have stereotyped ideas and images. They are likely to hinder the growth of imagination in a young child. Art is not for something, it is for itself. The process of creating a picture, for instance, is more important than the product, especially in childhood.

Assuming your son is 10 years old, I would say that a little bit of resistance to adult authority is quite normal. You can take care of it by spending time listening to your son to show that you are concerned about him and willing to give him your attention and affection. Ask him what he would like to do and gradually let him realize that working hard in any field is satisfying in itself.

Plan activities with him that you both enjoy. Don't focus only on drawing, but let him do it as he likes. He will ask for help himself. Suggest music or cricket or puzzles. If you take care of the child's interests now, you would be investing in his future. Happiness is the best tonic for mental and physical growth.

76. How do I handle my son who does not concentrate on studies?

Q. I have a 7-year-old son in class 2. He is harassing me a lot regarding his studies. He is very slow in writing and I have to go to his school or call up his classmates to take his work practically every single day. Today, he wrote only of 25 marks in a 50-mark, second terminal examination. I am really beating him up since he just does not listen. His teachers are complaining a lot too. It is not that he is dumb, he knows everything – even his teachers say so. He is very good in figuring out new gadgets etc. If not interrupted, he can watch TV for 8–10 hours and likes to play on the computer. He does not like to go out and play. What should I do?

A. Please stop beating your child! A child of 7 years is too young to be expected to sit for long hours and write fully. This is the age for playing and exploring the world. Do get him assessed by the school counsellor or any psychologist for reading or writing delay. He could also be suffering from an emotional problem such as oppositional defiance. You yourself acknowledge that he is intelligent. Try changing your handling of the child. Use positive encouragement and warmth. Physical punishment has not been found to be desirable in any way. It would only make him more defiant and escape into the safe world of television. He would develop a life-long aversion to studies and maybe even towards you!

77. How can I handle my daughter who is ignoring her studies?

Q. **My daughter is 5-and-a-half years old. I started working 2 months ago and now I find a change in her. She has started ignoring her studies and she starts crying when I try to make her study. She does not study easily and the class teacher says that she is easily distracted. She always needs my help and never tries to write on her own. I want her to concentrate more because she will soon be going to class 1. She has also started counter-questioning me. I can handle her coolly but at times when I am tired on reaching home, I lose my temper. She says that I am always scolding and hitting her. Please help me. I don't want to hit her but she is always crying for small things.**

A. It is important to understand that a 5-and-a-half-year-old child is not ready, physically or psychologically, to be put under undue stress of studies. You are perhaps not able to devote sufficient time and energy to her because of your job and your own stress could be making her demands appear difficult. Her problem seems to have started when you went to work. Her crying is a distress signal. Physically hitting or scolding the child will not produce desirable results. Try to schedule exclusive time with her when you are back from work. Make it a pleasant period. Try to show more patience, love and encouragement.

78. Why has the school labelled my child to have learning difficulty?

Q. **My 6-and-a-half-year-old daughter was said to have learning difficulty by the school. On questioning the principal, she was defensive and called my child a**

spoilt brat and an overconfident pampered child. My little one is a confident girl, helpful and sensitive to others. I am so disturbed that my sugar and blood pressure levels have shot up. Please help.

A. I can sympathize with your distress, but would also request you very strongly, not to be so upset. I agree that the principal should not have used such words to describe any child in her school. But sometimes, heads of schools get harassed with the demand for admission and for special treatment by parents who flaunt their wealth and social status. It is quite likely that she has had some unpleasant encounters with such parents and unfortunately put you and your child in the same category.

Perhaps, if it is feasible, you should consider changing schools. If that is not possible, you should make your peace with the school authorities and get on with life. Please find out if the child does have a learning difficulty. This is not a permanent condition and can be helped with the right kind of guidance. One of my friends calls it 'teaching disability' rather than 'learning disability'. But this is just a joke to cheer you up, which is not to be shared with the school! I do not know where you live. If you have access to a specialist, you could get your child assessed. There may be a few simple procedures to follow to help your daughter.

Most schools start reading and writing for children far too early. In the USA, children are 6-plus when they join first grade. They start reading and writing then. Here, in India, we tend to start writing in the KG classes. Most of us are victims of a badly planned school system.

Children need to have friends of their own age and many of them attend school only for that reason. Nevertheless, most children survive their dull classes to make something of themselves. Their natural resilience and energy serve as their best resource. You should not get so angry that it affects your blood pressure and sugar levels. Some exercises in Yoga could help you. Your own decision to stay calm and not to get upset will be the suggested treatment in this case.

79. My son feels bad about his handwriting, what should I do?

Q. My son is studying in class II and is 7 years old. His handwriting is very bad. On the first day of the new session, the teacher while introducing the students to the new teacher said in front of the whole class that his handwriting is very bad. On another occasion, one of his classmates also said, 'Oh! what a bad handwriting.' He was very hurt that day. When he

returned that afternoon, his friend told me about the incident. That day he kept asking, 'Mummy, is my handwriting so bad?' I soothed him by saying that we will do some homework and your handwriting will improve. In a few days it has improved a lot. Now another problem has erupted. He is learning 'maatras' in Hindi. They are learning 'OW'. During a class dictation, he made a number of mistakes, because he was still not clear about 'O' and 'OW'. He never got less than 80% in Hindi when he was in class I. Now in one dictation they have assessed that he is poor in Hindi and 5 of the children including my son have been asked to stay back in the class while others go for the music class. They may have done it for his benefit, but it hurts him a lot. He is too sensitive. During this one month, he has changed a lot and keeps thinking that he is useless. I don't know how to comfort him. Should I tell the teacher to allow him for music classes? Will it affect his future in anyway?

A. The two incidents you have reported are common occurrences in every school. Since your son's handwriting improved with a little attention, so will his use of Hindi spelling. There is no need to make an issue of it, in my view. The teacher can turn round and say, 'But my saying it has taken care of the problem!' You have to tell your son to be prepared for both praise and scolding. What you have narrated is not very sensitive on the part of the teacher, but not uncommon at all. The teacher was merely trying to achieve one immediate goal, i.e. to improve your child's Hindi.

Children are not as vulnerable as we think, but there is a vast difference in the way different children handle events of this kind and it is likely that your child is particularly sensitive. But instead of making it sound like a tragedy, you should say, 'Ah, you missed only one day's music class. You will soon catch up!' You could talk to the teacher and express some thoughts of course, but not instruct her on what to do. That kind of parental intervention is bound to be counter-productive. With children, we must be affectionate and empathetic. Adulthood gives you the advantage of objectivity and distance. Instead of getting affected every time he receives a remark or a punishment, be there for him, solid as a rock. That will take care of most problems. Ultimately, if a school system is found unsuitable for a number of reasons, study all possibilities and change schools. Convents were made for nuns, not for children!

80. Should I force my child to use his right hand?

Q. My son is 6 years old and in class II. He is left-handed and uses his right

hand only while eating. He is a slow child but he listens to what is taught in the class. The problem is with his handwriting, which is very bad. Moreover, sometimes he reverses the words. This worries me a lot. My husband and some of the teachers in class force him to use his right hand. And I am blamed for his left-handedness. Is it because of this problem that my child is not able to write the words properly? Please help me. ! find it difficult to take a 6-year-old child to a child consultant.

A. Ensure that your child is not forced to work with any particular hand. Let him have the freedom to choose. Handedness or the child's choice of hand depends on the wiring in the brain and forcing the child would simply frustrate him. You were right in letting him use the hand of his choice, but if he gets conflicting instructions, he will be confused. If his handwriting problems continue the next year, you should consult a child psychologist to rule out any learning disability. (*See also* page 72)

81. How can I handle my daughter who avoids studying?

Q. I have a lot of problems with my elder daughter regarding her studies. She doesn't copy anything from the blackboard. I have to go through her books everyday and call her friends to copy notes. Her excuse is that the teacher dictates very fast or writes very fast and erases the board; she is not able to cope up with her speed. She doesn't pay attention in the class. I have to take up all the lessons again every time she comes home saying that she doesn't know anything. She doesn't study on her own. I always have to push her to do her homework and study her lessons. She only wants to play with her sister. She goes to the toilet and sits there for half an hour to avoid studies. She takes a long time to finish her food. I am a working woman and I return home in the evening after which I have to cook food for my family. It is very difficult for me to handle her. I get tired and take out my anger on her by shouting and beating her. I have tried handling her with love and patience but it's of no use. How can I handle her?

A. You have given me a detailed report of your daughter without mentioning her age or class. The seriousness of her indifference to homework etc. will be defined by her age and class. Let me assume that your daughter is 10 years old and in class 4. There are two possibilities:

- She may not be at the level of a 10-year-old in her mental abilities. She may be finding school work difficult.

- She may be having some other problem due to which she is not able to attend to her lessons.

You will be the best person, having known her from her birth, which of the two explanations fits the situation. Please talk to her teachers and ask them what they suggest. You can give her a small specific job to complete and reward her with a hug or some praise if she does it on time and correctly. Keep repeating this procedure. Get the help of other members of the family, if they are available, so that you do not have to handle every problem yourself. See that the child is assessed by a psychologist or counsellor and make a proper plan for her education according to what she can do. You may need to be patient as she progresses gradually. Ask her what her reasons are for not taking homework down and do not assume that they are not true reasons. She may not only be troubling you - she may be troubled herself! Get the help of friends, neighbours and colleagues. Most people will be willing to help if there is a genuine problem.

82. Why does my husband not value education?

Q. My husband is a workaholic but, being a son of illiterate parents, he and my in-laws think hard work is more important. He does not worry about the daily homework of our children. This adversely affects them. How can children cope in this competitive world without having a good academic record? Please advise.

A. It is true that any extreme viewpoint is not healthy. But it is also a fact that attitudes differ between people in a single home! You as a mother would surely be able to inculcate desirable attitudes towards education in your children. You should do your best and not try too hard to change the other adults, as it would only create resentment. As the children grow up, they will analyse for themselves that education is important. If you think it is possible, try to meet a family therapist for suggestions and interventions.

Disciplining children

83. Why does my son throw tantrums only when he's with me?

Q. **My 6-year-old son is a quick learner, he grasps things very quickly and he loves to learn karate and watch action movies. He doesn't like to read and does not have friends as there are no children of his age in our area. Older children treat him like a kid and do not play with him due to which he beats them up. He is the only son. When at a relative's house, he is very obedient. My relatives say that he is a well-behaved boy and shows tantrums only when I am around. Please advise.**

A. Your son is an intelligent child as he is doing well at studies. Children get interested in storybooks if someone reads to them, while they follow the pictures in the book. You must have other books for him and he will develop a taste for reading. Try to talk to his teacher to understand the exact nature of the problem. Does the teacher expect too much from him or compare him with other children? If there is a school counsellor, it might be possible for you to discuss your child's behaviour with him.

Many children seem to have a good sense of where they can 'act up' and whom they can control through their behaviour. Parents often take the brunt of their children's aggression and discourtesy. They behave well at the homes of friends and relatives and soak in their approval. Maybe you need to change the way you handle him at home. An only child is usually pampered a lot. On the contrary, parents may have high expectations and can be very strict with the child. Try to study and understand your own handling of him. Children are playful by nature and do not always want to study or conform to school routines. Try to make him interested in different subjects. Praise him when he does homework on his own or writes well. Try not to compare him with others or criticize him or label him in a negative way. Encourage his strengths and be patient with his problems. (*See also* page 100)

84. How can I improve my daughter's 'nobody loves me' attitude?

Q. How do I help my 6-year-old daughter through her angry, hateful, 'nobody loves me' phase? She doesn't do anything and is full of sadness and anger. She screams and cries on everything I do. What should I do?

A. You must try to analyse the reasons for her behaviour.

- Has there been a change in the family scenario?
- Is there a medical problem with her?
- Are you over-indulgent with her?
- Do you give her adequate time and attention when she is in a positive frame of mind or does she only get attention when she misbehaves?
- As parents, are you role models of calmness or does she get to see aggressive behaviour?
- Are you sure that she has not been frightened or abused by anyone?

It is important to understand if her behaviour has changed suddenly or if she has been difficult since infancy.

On the whole, the best advice that can be given with the few details provided is that you should get her medically examined to rule out deficiency of any sort, worms, etc. Be good role models of behaviour yourself, and try to encourage her desirable behaviour and ignore negative behaviour, if possible. Spend time with her when she is playing with dolls, for instance, and listen to her. When she is relaxed, ask her gently why she is sometimes upset. It is unusual for a 6-year-old to feel that nobody loves her. Have you tried to see what the home is offering to make her feel that way? Perhaps there is a new baby in the house and the little girl feels that no one has time for her. Give her tenderness and some time, even if you have a busy schedule.

85. What can I do for my child who is perfect outside and the opposite at home?

Q. I am not sure where to begin. My 9-year-old girl came into the world

stubborn, but the trouble started 3 years back. She is wonderful in school, everyone likes her, and her teachers say she is a prized student. We feel very proud. However, when she is at home with her family, she is a nightmare. It is like she changes her personality when she gets in the car after school. I know it could be due to sibling rivalry, but this just does not seem normal. She says she hates me, or all of us, all the time. She starts arguments with all of us. She does not care what I, or her father, say about taking away privileges or sending her to her room. I am at the end of my rope. I have talked with the school counsellor and she was shocked. Who should I talk to and do you have any suggestions? We have done everything, from behaviour charts to spanking, but nothing seems to work. Others just can't imagine her behaving this way. I am worried since my other children (aged 4 and 7) too might take on the same behaviour. Please help.

A. You would definitely be having a hard time coping with a child who is perfect to the outside world and a difficult child at home. It is not easy to pinpoint the exact reasons for this difference in her behaviour, but since the problem started three years ago, it may be linked to either the birth of the youngest sibling or pre-adolescence.

Children these days are going through adolescent traumas earlier than before. A confusion in self-identity and a rebellious attitude at home are some of the indicators. My suggestion would be to get a complete psychological assessment done. She needs to be listened to very carefully to understand what themes underlie her stubbornness and defiance. The best alternative in dealing with her is to try to ignore her undesirable tantrums and negative comments. She is probably using them as attention-getting devices. On the other hand, try to give her adequate warmth and attention when she appears to be calm and in a good mood.

Finally, do remember that children go through phases. Hopefully she will come out of it soon. Try to be patient and serve as good role models yourselves.

86. My daughter takes a long time to wake up for school, what should I do?

Q. My 6-year-old daughter has been going to school since the age of 3. She never wakes up early. She takes a lot of time, cries, shouts, screams and wakes up after a lot of struggle. Even after waking up she takes about 25 minutes in the toilet. We keep telling her that she's getting late for school but she doesn't bother. If we make her understand things, she listens, but

repeats the same thing again. After all this, the only thing left is to scold her. I want her to understand these things; I have to explain everything to her. Otherwise, she is fine and a smart girl. Her teacher says that she is distracted in the class. She forgets what she did in class easily. Please guide.

A. Get your child assessed by a qualified psychologist or counsellor to rule out any attention deficit or cognitive problem. You must find out what happens in school and why she postpones going to it. Talk to her gently and let her tell you why she is unwilling to get ready for school. Children do find it hard to get up early in the morning to go to school but you should be firm and maybe wake her up even earlier to allow more time for the toilet. Also, make sure she goes to bed early and gets enough sleep. Reduce television watching and loud conversation at her bedtime. Ensure that you are good role models yourself and do not indulge in scolding or shouting.

87. How can I help my child become more aggressive in sports?

Q. My son is 9 years old and he doesn't enjoy contact sports. He wants to play basketball but during practice and games he doesn't get aggressive enough to go after the ball. He keeps his distance from the action. He just watches the game. He doesn't like to touch the football, instead runs away from the ball when it is thrown towards him because he is afraid of the ball. He is tall for his age and I have noticed that his shoe size is bigger than most of his friends. He is the slowest runner in his class. He gives up very easily and cries for everything. He is bright and loves video games and computers, but I limit it because I know he needs to exercise too. How can I help him become more aggressive and stop crying?

A. It is important to realize that children have different interests and temperaments. As a parent you should not force your child into any activity. Simply give him an opportunity to explore if it interests him and then decide if he wants to continue with it. If he feels frustrated he would not benefit and may develop a life-long aversion or fear for such situations. Your son seems to be shy and emotionally dependent. Try to encourage independent behaviour and ignore his crying. Let him take decisions and take responsibility for them. Emotional intelligence is as important as academic intelligence. You as a parent can help him by being supportive, firm and encouraging.

88. Are we neglecting our child?

Q. I have a 9-year-old son who is the second child out of our 4 children. He is always acting like he is 2 years old and tells other family members that he isn't allowed to eat or drink certain foods and that he doesn't have any toys. What should I do?

A. From your description, it seems to me that your son feels somewhat neglected among all his siblings.

Acting younger to one's age is quite common among children as a means of gaining their parents' or other people's attention. I am not sure how young your youngest child is, but it is possible that your son feels threatened by this new entrant and feels shortchanged in the bargain. Acting younger (2 years you say) makes him feel closer in age to the youngest sibling who, according to your son, is getting the attention that he wants for himself.

My suggestion would be to have a brief but reassuring talk with your son, letting him know that you care about him as much as you do about the other kids. Make him feel wanted and important. Make sure that he is included in family discussions and that his strengths are mentioned while talking about the other children. Find out if he behaves in a similar manner at school. Once he knows you love him as much as you love the others, this behaviour is bound to stop. If it continues for long, please consult a child psychologist.

89. Why does my daughter get distracted easily?

Q. My 8-year-old daughter is very talkative and gets distracted easily. How can I evaluate if she has an attention deficit disorder? A 5-minute task takes her 30 minutes. Right from brushing to dressing up for school, food habits, etc. are very time consuming. She does well when she concentrates. But her distractions ruin it all. She is good in her studies but that is also an extra effort. I want her to study for 30 minutes but she drags it to 1.5 hours. Her teacher has been complaining that she does not listen, keeps daydreaming and interrupts others sometimes. Her manners are very disappointing. Please advise.

A. Whatever label we give, the reality has to be handled. It does sound like your daughter can be easily distracted and does not concentrate on a task for more than a few minutes. Perhaps you should break up the jobs she has to do into smaller units. When she completes one, give her a pat on the back and let her go on to the next one. This would of course require your time and attention, but it may make it easier for her to focus. Sometimes good music (classical instrumental, Indian or western) can have a soothing effect, to calm her down. You will have to select the music carefully.

It is believed that TV, cola drinks and neon tubelights aggravate the situation for a child, who is prone to distraction. Encourage your daughter to read or tell a full story and listen to her so that she doesn't skip from one event to another. Make a game of her routine schedules, getting ready for school etc., and give her many chances to win. Be playful when dealing with her and she may start enjoying having you guide her.

Pick a sport in which she shows interest and let her take special lessons in it. Sometimes, even a game like ping pong will help the child to attend to detail and to coordinate her movements.

If your efforts do not have much effect even after a few weeks of these activities, you might wish to consult a psychologist or counsellor. Get your child interested in story books and she might get into the reading habit.

90. What is the reason for lack of concentration in my child?

Q. My 6-year-old son is not able to concentrate on anything. While eating, he just sits and keeps thinking of something. He has to be reminded again and again to eat. The same thing happens while he is studying or changing his clothes. We have to be after him continuously to get things done. If I ask him what happened in school after he returns, his standard reply is, 'I don't remember'. How can I tackle these things? Is it a problem of lack of concentration? Please suggest some games or toys to enhance his power of concentration.

A. You have not provided enough information for me to give you specific suggestions. For instance, what do the teachers say about your son? Is he interested in any toys, games or books? Does he have friends? Can he take care of his needs and be an active member of the family?

One way of enhancing the child's level of concentration is to see what he likes to do and then build upon that. I know a 7-year-old who was not too interested in maths. But when he started watching cricket, he could add or subtract scores mentally and remember a dozen details about every inning. His class performance has gone up. Perhaps, you as parents will have to make all his activities more interesting for him. As he eats, he could be told a story or you could plan something together, which he can enjoy after the meal. Songs and movements can be included. A moderate time (half an hour to an hour a day) in watching children's programmes on television could be a valuable addition to the stimulation.

Any of the common children's games available in bookshops can be used but according to the child's level. Even a pack of cards can become an educational tool, with the child learning to identify numbers and shapes. Talk to the child while you are doing things around the house and let him help you with small tasks that you assign. There is no simple formula for learning. We have to go by the child's temperament and inherent interests and abilities. We need to spend time with the child with affection and enjoyment and provide optimal stimulation for his mind to grow. Let the child get involved in playing with other children of his age. Children learn a great deal from each other. Be available for him when he needs support or has doubts about himself.

91. What should I do to handle a loud and talkative child?

Q. I have two children. One daughter – 9 years – is in standard IV and a son – 7 years – is studying in standard II. With the grace of the Almighty, they both are quite good in their studies and are quite attentive, adjusting and compassionate by nature. They are also well mannered. But I have one problem with my son. He speaks too loudly and too much. I mean he continuously talks, talks, and talks very loudly. The cause may be that when he was in nursery, his teacher told him to speak a bit loudly. Now he speaks loudly even when the listener is just near him. This situation creates a problematic scene at times. Kindly tell me how to tackle his problems of speaking loudly and speaking too much. I shall remain ever grateful to you.

A. Your problem does not seem to be very serious. However, you should try and find out why your son talks too loudly and too much. Is there anyone in the family that he imitates? Sometimes children do things to get the attention of their parents or other elders. If you assure him that you will listen even when he talks softly or in a normal way, he may talk like the others in the family.

Try making up a game, where everyone in the family will talk in whispers for half an hour. It will be enjoyable for your son to participate in the game and he will begin to see the advantages of talking softly. It will also be an opportunity for you to make sure that his hearing is all right. In cases where there is a hearing problem, children may talk too loud as they are not able to judge how loud or soft they are. This may not be the case with your child, but it is worth checking out.

You can also have a game where everyone in the family will communicate through writing notes to each other. For that period of 20 or 30 minutes, silence should be maintained. The novelty will make the children write better and also provide an alternative to speaking.

Plan activities (drawing, painting, music) for your children, which they enjoy as they learn and in which they can do well, without a sense of competition with each other. Do not compare the children, but treat them as individuals, with their own tastes and choices. Also try talking to your son directly, when he is relaxed and in a good mood, and tell him that you like it when he does not raise his voice. Also, listen to him carefully and respond, so that he gets the confidence of being listened to, even when he is not loud.

92. How can I make my girlfriend's children accept me?

Q. My girlfriend is a widow with two daughters of ages 7 and 10. Their father died in an accident 7 years ago. The children have had difficulties in accepting me. The younger one used to be very rude to me. I had the impression that this was instigated by the elder one, but she has improved over the past 3 months, although her rudeness recurs. The elder daughter is even more problematic. She is downright obnoxious and seems to want to goad me into getting angry and leave. Deep down, I feel that this is some sick game where she will win if I leave. Nine times out of 10, I do not react. Sometimes she feigns illness and pain in order to solicit her mother's attention, who gets very stressed. Today, she kicked me hard on the chin, drawing blood, and when I reacted angrily, she yelled blue murder and I felt like a child abuser. Her mother spoke to her about the incident later, but she denied kicking me. I have 3 grown-up children of my own, the youngest is still at school. I am divorced and my two young children live with me at home. The eldest has left the nest and supports herself. On the whole I feel they are stable, well-adjusted children. They think I am crazy for putting up with these monsters. My girlfriend and I get along very well and are enjoying our relationship. What can I do to improve the relationship with her children? Will they grow out of this behaviour?

A. I think that the child's mother must take an active part in socializing her daughters. They may harbour some resentment towards you and, therefore, be unlikely to pay attention to what you say. As you have sensed, the girls may think that they will have the mother to themselves if you were not in the picture. Therefore, it is her responsibility to talk to them at length and convince them that a joint home like yours can survive only when everybody observes the rules of courtesy and mutual consideration. If you are not able to handle this at home, there should be no hesitation in consulting a psychologist or a counsellor. A change for the better is possible, but would require some knowledge on how to handle the problem and patience on everybody's part.

93. How can I handle an obsessive and restless child?

Q. My son is 7-and-a-half years old. He is good in his studies. But I am worried about his behaviour. I feel he is hyperactive. He does not have friends. He makes friends easily but during play, he does something wrong thinking that it is also part of the game and loses them. It seems that he is not able to control himself. He can't sit quietly for 5 minutes. His class teacher also says he is restless. But when he is watching TV, he can sit for hours. If I watch another channel, he again becomes restless. He gets over-excited when guests come over. He is obsessive about food and thinks about food all day. During breakfast, he asks what will be served for lunch and dinner. He has a good diet. If I don't give him something to eat, he becomes violent. We go out for lunch/dinner once a week, but he wants to go out daily. Even when we are out in the market after lunch or dinner, he says that he is hungry and creates a scene in the market. Please advise.

A. Your query is incomplete and I am not sure what help you intended to ask for. If family routine for mealtimes had been established since childhood, perhaps he would not have developed an obsession for food. Since you have given no other detail about the members of the family and his interactions with them, I am not able to locate the root cause of his eating obsession.

You must get him interested in some active sport, where he can expend his energy and also excel. By now he should have started reading storybooks. You must plan more activities to occupy his time. Shopping and eating at restaurants do not constitute suitable leisure time activities for children of 7 years of age.

If you are not able to convince him that there are more worthwhile things to do than wait for the next meal, and to get him started on some new physical activity, try and consult a counsellor or psychologist who will guide you on how to proceed.

94. How should we deal with our son who does everything his own way?

Q. My 7-and-a-half-year-old son is very brilliant and is in grade 2. He has a good reading habit, grasping power and acute observance. He has a clear goal of becoming an astronaut since the age of 4. He hates being disciplined, especially while he watches TV or when it comes to being responsible for his own work. We are never harsh with him and allow him a certain time to watch TV, play games and do activities of his interest. He likes to do his school projects on his own, without any help. But once he sees that other students have done a better job, he gets disappointed. He is happy when we listen to him and do things his way but if we try to make him go the other way round, he becomes arrogant and stubborn. He demands toys and books whenever we go for shopping. We can't say no always, but don't want to say yes everytime. How should we deal with the situation?

A. Since your child is bright, explain to him that he has a choice:

- He can get help from the parents as other children do and have an error-free homework; or
- Do work his own way and be satisfied with it, even if other children's assignments are better.

Teach him to listen to you, just as you listen to him. If you can, do not constantly tell him he is brilliant and gifted. Talk to him about the values of being helpful, compassionate and kind. Old fashioned as they may sound, he will realize that they never get outdated. School systems put an emphasis on cognitive and mental achievement, even though societies and communities have more value for emotional intelligence. Cultivating both aspects would seem to be the road to wisdom.

Sex education

95. Is sexual inquisitiveness normal in young children?

Q. My 6-year-old son had a friend over for play. They went into his room and closed the door. Not hearing much from the room I became slightly suspicious. I entered the room to find my son lying on the bed with his pants lowered slightly. He looked guilty and said that his pants were falling down. My son had an erection too. I am not sure what the other child was doing or whether he was involved at all. Is this behaviour normal for a 6-year-old? Is it normal for a child to explore such things at such an early age? I am concerned and don't know how to deal with it. I think I should talk to the parents of the other child.

A. Sexual inquisitiveness is normal, and that in itself is not a problem. You should mention this to the parents of the other child. Both you and the second child's parents need to talk openly with your children. Ask them as to what was happening, and try and answer the questions in their minds. Give them honest answers based on their age and developmental stage. Do not scold or punish the children or make an issue out of this.

96. How should I handle a young child's curiosity about sexuality?

Q. The other day my 7-year-old son spent the night at my mother's home. She called me at 2 a.m. in the morning to inform me that she had woken up with him standing over her, naked. He had pulled off his clothes and straddled her leg and was rubbing his private part back and forth on her leg.

When she woke up, she asked him about his behaviour. We are not sure of how to deal with this. Please advise?

A. Your child must have observed a couple having sexual intercourse and must have become curious to see if he could do the same. One does not expect a 7-year-old to be so overtly imitative of the sexual act. I think your mother must have lost her nerve to call you at 2 a.m. to report it. There is something called infantile sexuality about which Sigmund Freud (psychoanalyst) and others have written extensively. Children realize that their private parts can be excited by touching or rubbing. They also realize that there is a lot of secrecy associated with sex and that adults will not answer their questions directly. They watch their parents and others in the home and draw their own conclusions. Little boys (and girls) will often say that when they grow up, they will marry a favourite aunt or a grandmother and have lots of children! It is still the age of innocence.

Your story about your son ended rather abruptly. I hope his grandmother did not punish him too severely. It is best not to make too much of it, while also conveying one's disapproval to the child. Other health aspects to look into would include reducing TV time and monitoring what the child sees. The food he eats should be bland and wholesome. The clothes he wears to sleep must be loose and light. Talk to the child patiently and also listen to him. Everything can be handled with maturity on your part. Let his father also talk to him, assuring him that when he grows up, he can act like a man.

97. Our daughter saw us having sex, what should we do?

Q. The other day my husband and I were having sex and our 8-year-old daughter suddenly walked into the room. Usually we are careful enough to lock the door, but last night we were so heated up that we forgot to lock the door. I tried speaking with her indirectly the next day, but she did not pay much attention. What was shocking was that I overheard my daughter's conversation with a friend of hers the following day. She was telling her friend that she enjoyed watching us do it and thanked her friend for giving the suggestion. I was shocked to hear the kind of details she was explaining to her friend! My husband has not taken this seriously but I am really worried. What should I do? I don't even know if I can discuss this with my daughter or the parents of this so-called friend?

A. All children are curious about sex, though not many of them from middle class families would have witnessed a sexual intercourse at the age of 8. For families that live in a hut or one-room tenement, it must be part of their daily reality.

Now that she knows so much, it is best to be candid and tell her that this happens among married couples and that young children should not talk or think about it and that they will grow up and eventually be involved in sex. If you have not told her how babies are made, this might be a good opportunity to tell her. You will not need the story of the birds and the bees.

Even if your daughter was egged on by a friend to enter your room, I don't think that much can be achieved by talking to the friend's mother. Almost all parents think that their ch ildren are innocent and simple, and it is their friends who mislead them.

Be direct and factual, not angry, when talking to your daughter. But advise her to be discreet and teach her to value privacy and confidentiality.

98. How can I tell my son about the birds and the bees?

Q. My son is 8 years old. He sleeps with us, as we are not interested to make him sleep separately because he is a single child. Although we are not engaged in sexual activities while he is awake, it seems that he is slowly developing curiosity about private parts. I would like to explain to him about the dos and don'ts, but have no idea how to start the conversation. What is the right age to tell him about the private parts and intercourse?

A. The best strategy for sex education of children is to answer their questions honestly and simply, using words and concepts that they can understand. This is the right age for you to introduce him to the male/female differences and to do so without undue embarrassment on your part.

Although you have not asked my view in this matter, I would like to advise you to have separate sleeping arrangements for your son. His being an only child is not a reason why he should be constrained to share his parents' room. Make it part of a birthday or new year present to him and let him savour the thrill of independence in his own bedroom, if you have the space. It is not that you are sending him out of your bedroom, rather that you are recognizing that he is growing up and would enjoy his own space.

Fears

99. How can I help my son get rid of his fears?

Q. My son (age 7) and my nephew (age 6) got spooked one night at a camp by some friends who thought they were being funny. Now they refuse to stay in a room by themselves (even if another child is there). It is becoming a huge problem. My son gets up 3–4 times at night. He sits on the toilet eating his cereal because he is scared to be in the kitchen alone, which is ten feet away. His fears are irrational to me, but totally rational to him. How do I help him without losing my patience?

A. Children at this age are fascinated by fantasy and have a wild imagination. The distinction between real and unreal is usually blurred. Your son has gone through a traumatic experience and is obviously very scared. He may overcome the fear on his own with time, but your patience and sensitivity in handling him are extremely important. Instead of criticizing him or belittling him, you should first of all provide a sense of security. Talk to him and let him express his true fears. Try to understand his reasoning even though you feel his fears are irrational. Explain to him that it was a prank and is to be taken as such. Encourage any small effort at moving away from fearful behaviour and try to ignore fear reactions. Give him deep breathing as an exercise. A chance to learn some Yoga may also be positive. If the family has religious inclinations, you could have him use prayers or chants to feel protected. You can also try using stories of courage and serving as a good example yourself.

10 to 13 year olds

- Shyness in children
- Help during divorce and separation
- Children and television viewing

- School issues
- Disciplining children
- Sex education
- Miscellaneous

Shyness in children

What is shyness?

Shyness is felt as a mix of emotions, including fear and interest, tension and pleasantness. It may lead to an increase in heart rate and blood pressure. Shyness can be a normal, adaptive response to any social experience. By being somewhat shy, children can withdraw temporarily and gain a sense of control. Generally, as children gain experience with unfamiliar people, shyness goes away. But if not, shyness can lead to problems such as:

- Less practice of social skills and fewer friends
- Poor self-image
- Low competence
- Less friendliness and likeability
- Children, who continue to be excessively shy, seem more lonely than their peers and have fewer close friends and relationships with members of the opposite sex in adolescence and adulthood
- At times, shyness may interfere with optimal social development and restrict a child's learning.

What are the causes for shyness?

The following may be the causes for shyness.

- Genetic.
- A not-so-firm bond between the parent and the child.
- Poor learning of social skills.
- Parents, siblings, or others, harshly and frequently teasing or criticizing a child.
- New social settings, especially if the shy person feels that he is the focus of attention is the most frequent cause of shyness.
- Some aspects of shyness are learned; a child's cultural background and family environment may offer such models of social behaviour.
- Sometimes the parents are too busy and are not able to meet the child's basic emotional needs by not spending enough time with him.
- Sometimes the child has an inferiority complex and feels inadequate in comparison to a sibling who might be smarter or better looking than him.
- Some children are timid by nature and seem to fear almost everything around them.

What can parents and teachers do to help children overcome shyness?

There are many strategies that can be used to help children overcome shyness. Some strategies may be more effective with some children than with others. The key is to recognize when a child's shyness is becoming a problem and then act accordingly.

- One way to help a child overcome shyness in certain social situations is to help him feel understood and accepted. Also, help the child identify and talk about his emotions. Let the child know that being shy is not a character flaw and it is nothing to be ashamed of.
- Prevent labelling the child as 'shy'. Children who are told that they are shy tend to start thinking of themselves as shy and stop making any effort to change.
- Set goals for more outgoing behaviour and then observe the child's progress. For many shy children, a realistic, challenging goal is to say at least one word to one new person every day. Other goals might include speaking in front of the whole class, or asking a question of the teacher.
- Set an example for the child. Children learn a great deal through observing the behaviour of parents and others. Parents who want their children to act in a more outgoing way should themselves act outgoing whenever possible in front of the children.
- Expose the child to unfamiliar settings and people. The more practice they get interacting with unfamiliar people, the faster the shyness will decrease. Prompt the child to interact with others.
- Reward the child for extrovert behaviour. For example, whenever he makes an effort to be outgoing, praise him.
- Help the child practice interacting with others. Some children do not know what to say in certain situations, such as when they meet a new child. Parents can help shy children by encouraging them to practice social skills.
- Accept the child and be sensitive to his interests and feelings. This can make the child more confident, less inhibited and also help build his self-esteem.
- Help the child develop social skills by providing him opportunities to experience social situations. For example, encourage the child to invite a friend or friends over to the house or to go over to a friend's house.
- Do not push a child into a situation which he considers threatening. Help the child feel secure and provide interesting material to help him participate in social situations.
- Share your experiences of being shy with the child.

Help during divorce and separation

Divorce is the termination of the family unit and, thus, it is often characterized by painful losses. Divorce and separation may be solutions to a discordant marriage, as they lead to decrease in hostility. However, for many children and their parents, tensions continue and the entire divorce process is a long, searing experience. For children, this process can be emotionally traumatic from the beginning of parental disagreement and rancour, through the divorce, and often for many years thereafter. Age-appropriate explanation and counselling is important, so that children realize that they are not the cause of, and cannot be the cure for, the divorce of their parents. Family guidance should be offered in dealing with children through the troubled time. They can be referred to professionals with expertise in the emotional, social, and legal aspects of divorce and its aftermath.

The divorce itself is usually not the only major change in the affected child's life. Children's sense of loss is ongoing and may increase, especially on holidays, birthdays, and special school events and when trying to integrate new family relationships. Other losses for the child or adolescent relate to changes in home, extended family, school, playmates, financial status, and parental work schedules. Up to 50% of children show a symptomatic response during the first year after their parents' divorce. Risk factors for continuing childhood difficulty include ongoing parental discord, maternal depression, psychiatric disorders in either of the parents and poverty. Long-term follow-up studies indicate that divorce may limit or delay children's capacity for intimacy and commitment as young adults.

Children's reactions

The clinical manifestations of divorce in children depend on many variables including the child's age; the pre-divorce level of the family's psychosocial functioning; the parents' ability to focus on their child's feelings and needs in the middle of their own anger, loss and discomfort; and the child's temperament and temperamental fit of parents with their children.

Infants and children younger than 3 years may reflect their distress, grief, and preoccupation. They often show irritability, increased crying, fearfulness, separation anxiety, sleep and gastrointestinal problems, aggression and developmental regression.

At 4–5 years of age, children often blame themselves for the break up and parental unhappiness, become more clingy, show externalizing behaviour (acting out), misperceive the events of the divorce situation, fear that they will be abandoned, and have more nightmares and fantasies.

School-aged children may be moody or preoccupied; show more aggression, temper, and acting-out behaviour; seem uncomfortable with gender identity; and feel rejected and deceived by the absent parent. School performance may drop, and they may agonize about their divided loyalties and feel that they should be punished.

Adolescents may feel low in self-esteem and may develop premature emotional autonomy to deal with negative feelings about the divorce. Their anger and confusion often lead to relationship problems, substance abuse, decreased school performance, inappropriate sexual behaviour, depression, aggressive and delinquent behaviour.

Children of all ages frequently have psychosomatic symptoms as a response to anger, loss, grief, feeling unloved, and other stressors. They may try to play one parent against the other because they need to feel in control and test rules and limits. However, they are likely to feel guilty and responsible for the separation and feel that they should try to restore the marriage.

Parents' reactions

Parents also suffer detrimental effects from divorce and manifest a variety of negative and uncomfortable reactions. Mothers are likely to react to daily stressors as well as to the untoward major event in the following ways: consume more alcohol, use more mental health services for depression, anxiety, or feelings of humiliation, and to feel overwhelmed and less capable as parents. Fathers often feel pushed away, are likely to seem less accepting of their children, and also may develop depression, anxiety, and substance abuse. Grandparents as well often perceive a decreased quality of relationship with their grandchildren, with custody arrangements being more influential in determining visiting schedules than is geographic distance.

How can doctors assist children and families?

- Be alert to warning signs of dysfunctional marriage and impending separation.
- Discuss family functioning in anticipatory guidance and offer advice pertinent to divorce as appropriate.
- Always be the child's advocate, offering support and age-appropriate advice to the child and parents regarding reactions to divorce, especially guilt, anger, sadness, and perceived loss of love.
- Paediatricians must try to maintain positive relationships with both parents rather than taking sides. If there is evidence of an abusive situation, referral to child protective services should be indicated.

- Encourage open discussion about separation and divorce with and between parents, emphasizing ways to deal with children's reactions and identifying appropriate reading materials.
- Refer families to mental health resources with expertise in divorce, if necessary.

Long-term follow-up

Although many children have long-lasting emotional and adjustment problems associated with their parents' divorce, most adjust and function well over time, particularly those who have supportive relationships and a positive temperament and receive professional counselling.

Substantive periods of change during the process can demand new adjustments on the part of the children. Although the legal divorce is an important event for parents, it may be an insignificant event to a younger child who knows little of the legal process or a very significant event for the older child who experiences further proof that his parents will not reconcile. Parents' dating and sexual activities may be troublesome for children. Parental discretion and truthfulness are important for maintaining respect for the parents. Step-families may pose another adjustment challenge for the children and their parents. As children develop and mature, their emotions, behaviours, and needs with regard to the divorce are likely to change. A custody arrangement that made sense for a younger child may need adjustment for a preadolescent or adolescent. With their advancing maturity, awakening sexuality, and important steps towards their own adulthood, their parents' divorce is reinterpreted and requires re-discussion and readjustment. Many behavioural and emotional reactions from the separation can be reawakened at times of subsequent loss, at anniversaries, with the child's advancing maturity, and with the need to adjust to new and different family structures.

Children and television viewing

A child sitting with a remote of what is popularly called the 'idiot box' could watch anything from cartoons to programmes with murders and sexual content that is not suitable for young minds. Television characters are often exaggerated stereotypes that can distort children's expectations of people in day-to-day life. Topics such as drug abuse, alcoholism, and sex may also be brought to the child's attention sooner than necessary. In addition, children often have trouble distinguishing fantasy from reality on TV.

There are potential benefits from viewing some television shows, for example learning positive aspects of social behaviour such as sharing and cooperation, but TV viewing can also result in many negative health effects. Research shows primary negative health effects are on aggressive behaviour, sexuality, academic performance, body concept and self-image, nutrition, dieting, obesity, and substance abuse. Children and adolescents are particularly vulnerable to the messages conveyed through television, which influence their way of thinking and behaviour.

Violence on the screen

People have blamed the television for children throwing themselves off the roofs or risking their lives doing dangerous stunts in an attempt to copy superheroes and models in advertisements. Some even believe that brutality on television could be the direct cause for juvenile crime. Programmes that show huge wrestlers fighting with each other to excite a screaming public and even seemingly innocuous cartoons such as *Tom and Jerry*, where they are seen constantly bashing each other, send certain messages to children. Through such violent programmes, children get the idea that violence is a means to power. The three major effects of viewing TV violence are:

1. Children may become less sensitive to the pain and suffering of others.
2. Children may be more fearful of the world around them.
3. Children may behave in an aggressive or harmful way towards other people.

Parents can limit the effects of violence by observing the following:

- View TV together and discuss the violence with the child. Talk about why the violence happened and how painful it is. Ask the child how conflicts can be solved without violence.
- Explain to your child how violence on an entertainment programme is actually 'fake'.
- Restrict violent videos.

- Encourage your child to watch programmes with characters that cooperate, help, and care for each other. These programmes have been shown to have a positive influence on children.
- Read to your child rather than watching television. Stories meant for children and written by thoughtful authors portray conflict in a more realistic and constructive manner.

Monitoring television viewing

Children are very impressionable and it is important to monitor what they view. Paediatricians recommend the following guidelines for parents.

- Limit the duration of TV viewing by children to 1–2 hours of quality programmes per day.
- Do not provide television sets in their bedrooms.
- Discourage television viewing for children younger than 2 years, and encourage more interactive activities, such as talking, playing, singing, and reading together.
- Monitor the shows that children and adolescents view. Most programmes should be informational, educational, and non-violent or programmes which demonstrate helping, caring and cooperative behaviour.
- View television programmes along with children, and discuss the content. Two recent surveys involving a total of nearly 1500 parents found that less than half of the parents reported that they always watch television with their children.
- Set a weekly viewing limit. At the beginning of the week, have your child select programmes appropriate for her.
- Rule out TV at certain times such as mealtimes and sleeping hours.
- Remember that children learn from their parents. If you watch a lot of TV, the chances are your child will do the same.
- Parents should work out a timetable for watching television with their children.
- Discuss with your child what is real and what is make-believe on TV. Explain how television uses stunt actors, camera zooms, dream sequences and animation to create fantasy.

What is a good quality programme?

Parents differ in the ways in which they assess the quality of a programme, but they are the best judge of what they consider to be suitable for their child. However, there are some general rules that you might use in selecting programmes which you would encourage your children to watch. Television is most effective as a teacher when it is in tune with the needs of the viewer. For children, the best programmes are those that speak to them in ways they can understand about topics that are important to them.

Also, good programmes encourage children to explore their feelings, learn about their world, and increase their competence and self-worth. Those that exploit children's feelings of envy, competitiveness and anger, or encourage narrow and stereotyped views of the world, do not help children to grow and develop. Good programmes do not need to be 'educational' in the sense of being designed to instruct children. Rather, the best TV-teachers are entertaining, informative and child-centred and expand the horizons of the young minds. (*See also* page 182)

School issues

100. How should we parent a stubborn child who lacks interest in studies?

Q. This is regarding my son who will turn 12 this year. We have noticed a very arrogant streak and some behavioural changes in our child especially when it is time to study. He studies for a short time and then gets restless. If we beat him he becomes violent and dangerous, and hits back. He does not like to be beaten and hence we cannot correct his behaviour. Last year, he fell from the cycle and got a big lump at the back of his head, which subsided later. A scan of the head was done and the report was normal with no skull injury. He only wants to enjoy life and rest, and take life easy. Please let me know if he should be taken to a psychiatrist? A few months ago, in school, he had a black out with acute pain in the head and could not see anything. He slept with his head on the desk for a few minutes and then was fine. He is thinly built and is very fussy about food. He is excellent at playing video games, chess and football. What should we do?

A. Dear parents, I think you are interested in your son doing well in school, so that he can have a happy and successful future. But in the process, you are making it very hard for him to be happy or successful in the present. Let me explain.

He has had a head injury 8 months ago and a blackout a month ago. Perhaps it has not occurred to you that his minor behavioural problems could be a result of the injuries. I use the word minor deliberately. Nothing that you have reported suggests a major problem, except perhaps in your perception of your son. He enjoys video games and chess, you say. That indicates a good level of brain functioning. He enjoys football with his neighbours, you say. That is a clear indication of appropriate social functioning. I find that you are very severe in your judgement of him. By treating him as you do, it can be expected that he will get angry and retaliate.

Why should you beat a child? Give him a little more psychological space. Let him take responsibility for his own work, without the nagging presence of parents. If he gets pulled up in school, he will learn to pay more attention and to complete his assignments. Surely, being playful as an 11-year-old cannot be a crime!

Children of this age are gradually outgrowing their childhood and would not like to be under an autocratic regimen, in school or home. A little gentleness and humour on your part will certainly help. Share some of his interests with him. You say that he does not like to be beaten (slapped). Do you know anyone who likes it? We as adults use our power and authority over children to arrive at some goal that we have set. Each child is unique and individual in interests and inclinations. There is no standard mould into which they must fit. If you continue to be so harsh, your child will submit for the time being and then get away as soon as he can. Your child is given to you in trust (Khalil Gibran has a beautiful verse about it). Use your parenting years more enjoyably.

101. Is my child in an age appropriate class?

Q. My child is 10 years old but she is in the 5th standard. Is this age appropriate? We got her admitted at the age of 3 years and 2 months instead of 3-and-a-half years in a playgroup. Now, I am a bit disturbed about her maturity and grasping power. Someone suggested to me to get her a one-year gap. Is this preferable?

A. It is not unusual for a child to be in a class where she is a few months younger than the others. If she has adjusted, it may be best to leave her there. She may face a problem with taking a gap year. She might feel bad about failing and also losing out on her friends. In case you find that she is not able to cope with increasing workload, then you may consider a change of class or even a change of school. Do ask the child's opinion before you consider any major change. Her teachers may also be able to give you the right advice.

102. Why do I forget everything just before the exams?

Q. **I am 12 years old, studying in the 9th grade. I perform well in class but fail to perform well during examinations. I feel really depressed when I get my results. As of now I have reached the 9th grade but I don't want to get bad results. I don't know why this is happening? My teachers have been complaining since I was 9 years old. I really feel bad when everyone advises me to study well. I really work hard and remember everything before the exams but after seeing the question paper I forget everything. I also want to gain weight since I look like a skeleton.**

A. You seem to suffer from examination anxiety. You need to learn stress management techniques, such as deep breathing and time management. Do not study too much just before an exam. Start preparing for the exam ahead of time. Try to learn the lesson in short points after understanding. When sitting for an exam, take deep breaths before reading the question paper. Spend 2 minutes to read the paper well. Tell yourself that you can answer well. Stop repeating to yourself that you do not remember anything. Start writing any answer that appears to be easy. Take one step at a time. You will soon find that you are able to tackle all the questions well. If you do not improve, consult a psychologist or medical doctor.

The simplest way to add to your body weight is to eat more. Have nutritious snacks, mid-morning and before bedtime. If that is not possible, increase the amounts you normally eat. Eat with enjoyment and tell your family how good it tastes. Spend time outdoors and have lots of activity. Check with your doctor whether you need de-worming and take the necessary pills only under his advice and guidance.
(*See also* page 190)

103. Will my child, with learning difficulties, be able to graduate?

Q. **My son is 10 years old. He has learning difficulties; we had tested his IQ, which was found to be 58 with minor difficulties. Now, with age he has improved a lot but his speech is still not clear. He cannot defend himself against others, cannot make words on his own, and is very poor in studies and misses many words. He gets about 60% marks with a lot of effort. I want to know whether there is any scope for him to improve? Will he be able to complete graduation in any field or not? Will he become mature enough and face the outside world? Please help me. I am also very worried about the**

size of his penis which is very small as compared to other children even below his age. Is this too because of his low mental development? Do I need to consult some doctor?

A. It is hard to predict whether your son will be able to complete graduation, as it would depend on the amount of enrichment and special education provided to him. It would be better for you not to have very high academic expectations from him. Excelling in studies is not everything in life. He must be having some special talents. Try to identify and build on those. He is too young to be sexually mature. Do keep in touch with special educators, speech therapists and clinical psychologists.

104. Should we force our child to stop playing and study all the time?

Q. We have one son, 11 years, studying in the 6th standard. He is very good at studies and mostly scores above 90% with 2nd/3rd rank in the class. I am a working professional whereas my spouse is a housewife. My son is very fond of playing with his friends besides playing computer games at home. My wife keeps on objecting to his playing any game and tries to demotivate him. She always irritates him by stopping the play. If I intervene she alleges that I am spoiling his future and this creates a lot of trouble and tension. My son is also very demanding and aggressive. He will never give up his demands. If you force him then he won't eat food. Further, my wife teaches him at home, except maths, which I teach him. Kindly suggest how to tackle this problem.

A. You are right in not wanting to force your son unnecessarily. He is already doing well at school, but is his performance at school mainly due to the mother's hard work with him? Your wife may be having unrealistic and high expectations from him. He is approaching adolescence and it is important not to force or nag him, but use reasoning and discussion to arrive at mutually acceptable standards. There is some truth in the old adage, 'All work and no play makes Jack a dull boy'. When a child is doing well in his school, it seems unnecessary to push him towards more achievement. A balanced schedule including work and play is the best option.

105. Will my child be able to cope with studies?

Q. I am a mother of an 11-year-old girl. From early childhood, she's been

having problems at school regarding her studies. Now that she is in standard 6, she has failed in 5 subjects in her 1st term exams. Her school teacher has advised me to take her for counselling. What effect will this have on the child? Will she be able to cope with the CBSE standard of education? What are the rules of these institutions? Will they detain her this academic year?

A. If your child has found it difficult to cope with her studies, it would be better if she were in a less demanding system. CBSE is by far too heavy in the curricular load, for most children. It might be a good idea to take her teacher's advice and see a counsellor. This will help you and the child to have realistic expectations. There will be no adverse effect on the child. A counsellor will only test the child and let you know how to proceed with her education. I have no idea about the school she attends, so I cannot answer your question about rules. If they detain her, you might continue her in the same school for the next year. It will give her time to catch up with the subjects that were difficult earlier. If she has interest in music, art or dance, you might give her an opportunity to pick up those skills. It is also possible for her to shift to the Open School system and take a few exams at a time in the subjects of her choice. I know of many children who have been helped by this alternative system.

106. How can I handle my son's reading problems?

Q. My son is 10 years old. I am concerned about his reading speed. He seems to be a very slow reader. Observing his slowness as compared to his peers, I had put him in a reading programme last year. Since then, he has made some improvement, but not to match with the average children of his age. I have made the following observations – many times he reads 'b' as 'd' and 'd' as 'b' and loses track of the sentences once he realizes his mistake. He gets confused whether to use 'c' or 'k' sound for words involving ce, ca, ci, cu, etc. Often, he reads 'is' as 'in' and 'then' as 'when', etc. When I ask him to spell out longer words, which he cannot read, he spells wrongly, e.g. C as S, H as T. He's good at mathematics. He can solve arithmetic problems up to his grade level. He can also solve all logical problems pretty well. Please advise.

A. I must congratulate you on the detailed observation you have made of your son's reading abilities and errors. From what I can see, he seems to have dyslexia, which is not uncommon and does not continue to be a problem. If you have access to a psychologist or counsellor in the place you live, a consultation might help. However, here are some general words of advice. Do not compare him with other children. He may be good at drawing or music or football. If he is, emphasizing the strengths will also help him. Finally, all children get interested in reading once they read stories. Comprehending a story is the motivation (and spelling or pronouncing is only incidental)! Silent reading is the best way to make a child read a lot.

Dyslexia is something that seems to largely disappear as the child grows older. Major cities in India have some professional organizations to help children with dyslexia.

107. Why is my son not able to write down the answers he knows?

Q. My son is 10 years old and weak in studies. But my daughter is clever. My son studies in standard 5 and my daughter studies in standard 1. The problem with my son is that he is able to say all the answers, but he is not able to write the same. Is this a medical problem?

A. If your son is 10 years old and is studying in standard 5, I do not think that he has a medical problem.

Schools usually give a lot of writing work, but not all children like to write. Some cannot write. Does your son like to read? Does he have friends? Does he talk to you about what he does in school? Do his teachers like him? If the answer to these questions is 'yes', the problem can be taken care of with just a little attention.

It would be a good idea to consult a psychologist or school counsellor to get an idea of what methods would work best for him. I don't want to suggest that there is anything wrong, but I would need more details to know what exactly to tell you.

Also, consider the strengths of the child. Perhaps he is good in sports. Possibly he has a talent for music. Maybe he draws very well or tells jokes and keeps everyone laughing. Find out what his strong points are and let him know that he is appreciated for them. Then start working on his writing. He will pick up skills as he grows up. Try not to compare the two children. Each child has something to offer to you and to the family.

Disciplining children

108. How can I tackle my children who are careless about hygiene?

Q. My 12- and 10-year-old sons are very reluctant to use soap during their bath. I have tried giving them rewards and changing soaps, but no use. Brushing teeth is another problem for them. They seldom comb their hair unless I force them to do so. Please advise.

A. I know boys sometimes place no importance on personal hygiene, but I haven't heard of such adamant loyalty for the natural state and such disdain for the niceties of civilization! Surely there are rules at school too. Can the teachers not help in this process? What about the father?

There are some suggestions you can try. You can give your sons a choice of being totally bald (which you will see is done if they do not wash their hair regularly) or taking showers and using shampoo, etc. Show them how terrible it is to be in the same room with unwashed people by making them smell a dead lizard or a dead rat. Ask them if they want to be shunned by their friends. Once a week, you could give them a bath and show them all the major steps. Instead of offering new soaps, you might think of something to play with or to eat as a reward, which they will really appreciate.

Also you could refuse to serve them dinner unless they are properly bathed. One evening's starvation will not be so difficult. But let them not substitute dinner with junk food that they can buy. Be firm with them, while also showing that you care. (*See also* page 101)

109. How can I prevent my 10-year-old son from telling lies?

Q. How to prevent my 10-year-old son from telling lies? We are working parents and neither of us tell lies or encourage the child to do so (like while attending phone calls). We tell him all kinds of moral-based stories. One of us does not believe in hitting/whacking and always softly inculcates the value while the other takes to hitting for grave mistakes. But we find he lies, rather fibs, and every time gets caught. There has never been any complaint at the school or at other places. We have also told him that whatever be the mistake, he would not be punished and he can confess – so that the fear of punishment would not be there in him and he tells the truth. We are concerned if he is into compulsive lying. We are friendly with him and discuss various subjects in a healthy environment. Where have we gone wrong? Or are we unduly worried?

A. I think it is important to examine the kind of lies your son tells and the issues around which they occur. Is there a point to his distortion of the truth? For example, if he says that there is no homework that might be a lie to save him from working on it. But if he makes up stories which would be of no benefit to him, it is a different situation. So, instead of putting all lies into one category, try and study which events or episodes lead to lying.

When you have discovered that he is not speaking the truth, have you asked him the reason or just punished him? The more we explain our rules, as well as our punishments, to the child, the more likely it is that he will learn to abide by your rules. There are some children who may do something wrong to get the attention of the parents. Make sure that you give him time and affection when he is well behaved, so that being noticed for being naughty is no longer a reward.

The key to the problem is to find out why he prefers to mask the truth. Beating him may not have a positive effect at all. At 10 years of age, he can think and reason and your treatment of his behaviour should recognize and reflect that fact.

Sometimes, children tell their friends that they have 6 cars at home. This may be done by a child to impress his friends and make them respect him! The strategy usually fails.

Although you ask him to speak the truth and promise nothing will happen, it appears that you do beat him after that. You must keep your word so that he learns to trust you. If his behaviour at school is all right and it is only at home that he lies, don't you think that you have to make sure that you are not confusing him and somehow making the home, the problem? Things can be worked out, but do give it your close attention and try to be consistent. (*See also* pages 84, 101)

110. My child feels ashamed that we are not financially well-off, please help?

Q. Ours is a middle class family with both my wife and I working. My two children are in the care of my parents till 6 p.m. We have been able to admit our elder daughter in a reputed Delhi school and she is in standard 5. Most of her classmates are children of rich businessmen or senior government officials. Of late, she has been complaining that her friends tease her about her financial background, few of her friends who have visited our small flat, have told others that my daughter stays in a small house and her parents are not financially well-off, though I have given my children an above-average standard of living and amenities. My daughter, otherwise, is a bright and active student, but now, quite regularly, she rakes up the above issue. Please advise me on how to make my daughter understand and handle the situation?

A. Your daughter's problem is not uncommon. Children tend to compare themselves with each other. Some children, who may be from families that are newly rich, try to establish that they are superior because they are rich. This is not true, of course. You should tell your daughter that it is important to be a nice, helpful and kind person and to be a good student who is interested in learning new things and willing to share both time and knowledge. I have taught generations of students and can tell you that these qualities (along with a sense of humour) are the qualities that are most liked.

Showing off about being richer is something that will disappear as the children become more mature. You should tell your child that the great success stories in our own times are those of people with humble beginnings and who worked hard. Our President, Abdul Kalaam, grew up as a boat-maker's son and studied on scholarships, and our Prime Minister, Manmohan Singh, is from a simple farming family. See where they have arrived and how much respect they command around the world. You must feel convinced about true values and tell your daughter not to bother about petty comments from her classmates. Since you mention that it is a reputed school, you could also talk to her teachers and have them establish the right values in the school.

Finally, some of these things will not go away and your daughter will have to develop her own methods to deal with them. Also, request the others in the family to help you in dealing with this.

111. How should I handle my stepson's stealing problem?

Q. I have been married for the past 5 years. My husband is a very loving and caring person. He has two children from his ex-wife and now we have a child together. He is a kind man, who believes that his children can't do anything wrong. Once I approached my husband about our second son's stealing habit, but he didn't believe me. He becomes upset when I accuse our son of anything and feels that I just keep blaming him. I can't talk to his ex-wife because she and my husband are not on talking terms. Recently, a note of Rs 100 was stolen from my safe keeping spot and I found that our middle son was acting very strange. He has a history of stealing since the age of 6; when he opened a birthday gift addressed to a friend's daughter and stole the glitter from the box and hid it in the bathroom. I always find the evidence of things he has stolen in his bag or drawer. Now he is trying to blame his 3-year-old brother. My husband is upset with me and says that I am making our son feel like an outcast. What should I do?

A. Your concern about your stepson is understandable. But perhaps you need to change the way of dealing with the concern and the information that you have. This would involve changes in two aspects: your dealing with the child and your sharing the concerns with your husband.

Telling your husband directly would make him feel defensive as he may feel you are acting like a typical stepmother. The best way would be let him understand that you are the child's well-wisher and unbiased.

Showing positive gestures whenever the child shows desirable behaviours would help in dealing with the child and also would convince the father about your fairness and genuine concerns. Try to form a rapport with the child. Discussing and reasoning are always more effective than blaming and scolding. Unconditional warmth and setting of limits would prove useful with the child. Maybe it is difficult, but you should start thinking of them as your children, not as 'stepchildren'. If a 6-year-old child took some 'glitter' from a box, I would not term it as having a history of stealing. A little more warmth and a sense of humour could take care of most problems. If these strategies do not work for you, you may like to consult a psychologist or counsellor about your children.

112. How can I fill in the place of a missing father figure in my daughter's life?

Q. I am a 36-year-old widow having a 12-year-old daughter. My husband died when my daughter was a month old. I had many ups and downs, which I dealt with normally. Suddenly I feel that my daughter is missing a father figure in her life. She has been away from a male figure as I have been staying alone. I have also kept her away from my male friends, which has been a better way to deal with things. She has been a very good child, but I am not sure if I have been a good mother to her. I have been working all these years and have been busy in handling my emotions and myself. What best can I do for my daughter? What should I do, so that she doesn't become emotionally vulnerable at this age, especially when she is about to be a teenager? I want to provide her with all the emotional comfort and would like to make her emotionally strong and independent. Is it right to do so or am I expecting too much from her?

A. You seem to be dealing with a lot in your life indeed, and you are managing it well too. One must appreciate that you are so concerned about the psychological health of your daughter. Adolescence is a very important stage of development, which not only involves physical changes, but also mental and emotional changes. It is a stage of confusion for most teenagers as they are unable to make sense of the ongoing changes in their body and manage their relationships. Patience, understanding and communication are the three key words to deal with an adolescent.

My advice to you would be to talk to your daughter and try to ascertain if she has concerns regarding the lack of a father figure in her life. A grandfather, an uncle, a teacher in school, a male friend of yours - any one of these can serve, to some extent at least, as a father figure. Adopt a friendly approach towards her and listen to her. Answer her questions. Prepare her for puberty and the beginning of sexuality. Give her certain responsibilities to be handled independently and appreciate her for her efforts. A balance between parental control and giving independence needs to be maintained. Also, make the best decisions for your own life and career and as long as she has your love and care; she will adjust to them. Emotional strength comes from trust and mutual affection.

113. How to handle an only child who lacks maturity?

Q. **I have a 10-year-old son. He is very playful, childish and sweet but sensitive. Being an only child, he wants attention and is moody. He lacks the maturity that we see in other children of his age. He lacks confidence and is totally dependent on me. There is a lot of anger in him, which he says he cannot control. He seeks our approval all the time. His way of talking and behaving is very childish. He is still a baby in his mind. Please tell me how to handle him?**

A. An only child can show dependency and immaturity, as he or she is the subject of total adult attention. The child becomes afraid of criticism and, therefore, avoids independent responsibility. To deal with your son's problems, encourage his efforts at independent thinking and working. Avoid criticisms and try to teach him anger management skills, especially by giving your own example.

114. How can we help our daughter deal with new surroundings?

Q. **My 11-year-old daughter studies in an English medium school. We have recently shifted to a new city. She is having difficulties in interacting with her classmates. She wants to get along with them but they don't entertain her. She is gradually withdrawing in her own self and losing self-confidence, which is slowly reflecting in her results. Her teachers don't have any complaints against her. She quarrels a lot with her younger brother. We are unable to handle this. Please advise.**

A. Early adolescence can be a difficult time for most children, and for your daughter it is even more complicated with drastic changes in city, school, friends and medium of instruction. Give her some time to adjust to the new situation.

As a parent you can also take certain steps:

- Talk to her and listen to her. Spend time doing interesting things with her.
- Show your unconditional love, acceptance and support for her.
- Keep in touch with her new teachers and make them aware of her problems.
- Encourage her to make friends, but do not force her or criticize her if she does not take initiative.
- Get professional psychological help, if required, from the school counsellor.

115. Is our marital discord affecting our daughter?

Q. **My husband and I argue a lot. He even tends to verbally abuse me and says vile things. Our 10-year-old daughter has been hearing our arguments all her life. I have noticed that she is becoming anxious and rather demanding towards my husband and me. She treats me as if I don't know what I am talking about. She does not let her father get away with saying bad things to me. I am not sure what to do. Do you recommend any books or do you think she needs counselling?**

A. It seems as though your 10-year-old daughter is more mature than her parents. She is absolutely right in stopping your husband from using abusive language towards you. You should have kept her out of the scene, while you were arguing. At least now, avoid acrimonious scenes when the child is around. It is also possible for both of you to go to a marriage counsellor for advice on how to manage your relationship. When the family is peaceful and harmonious, the girl will definitely be less anxious. Please take the message that the girl is giving to you both: let's have peace and warmth in my home.

116. My son needs to be pushed for doing everything, what should I do?

Q. **My son is 12 years old. He is very fast in doing tasks allotted to him. But he doesn't get up early in the morning and we have to force him to get up for school. He gets up with a reluctant mind coupled with shouting at his parents for forcing him to rise early. But once he is up, he gets ready very fast and has missed the school bus only once in 8 years. He goes off to sleep only around 11 p.m. What should I do? Secondly, I have been doing yoga for the past 7 years. I have tried all means to persuade my son to do yoga, at least once or twice a week. But he has an aversion towards this age-old magic. When I see other children of his age doing yoga, I feel sad. Also, many children of his age do household chores with joy. But my son does a few household chores and that too with reluctance. Regarding studies, he is good and scores 85% or so. But we have to be after him for studying. He is fond of playing cricket, watching TV and playing computer games. He cycles occasionally. He eats a fair quantity of fast food such as pizzas, patties, etc. He is overweight. Please advise.**

A. It seems as if you are part of the conspiracy to keep your son doing all the things that you disapprove!

To start with the last point first. Refuse to let your son have fatty foods all the time. Restrict it to once a week. He should not be allowed to do whatever he likes. Your authority should be firm. But since you have allowed such behaviour for months, all your work with him will have to be slower now.

Get him into a group that plays active games. Make the exercises also enjoyable. Yoga is somewhat solitary and may not be attractive to all children.

If he can get 85%, he should be challenged to do even better, not necessarily with school marks, but in mastering some other skill. Have you tried karate, for instance? Let his cycling become more regular. Encourage him by saying that if he wishes to be a part of the Commonwealth Games, he will have to begin now!

You could also refuse to drop him at the school bus and see if he makes it on his own. He is trying to push his limits and you are giving in each time. In the old days, there was scouting as a movement and children who were scouts became helpful and cooperative as well. Try and locate such a group which encourages activity and a helpful attitude.

I find it surprising that you are sad at what he is doing. You could get happy by being more firm and being consistent. Try and rope in his favourite uncle or teacher to help you plan the details of the strategy.

117. How can I make my daughter respect her elders?

Q. My daughter is 12 years old and has a bad habit of lying with finesse. Recently, she has become very arrogant and has even gone to the extent of slapping her grandmother who has take care her since her birth. I do not understand her ways. My wife and I have tried to talk to her, explained situations and also scolded and beaten her at times, but to no avail. This recent behaviour of raising her hand on her grandmother has brought a lot of unrest in the family. How should we go about this?

A. I think your concern is realistic. Why would a 12-year-old hit her grandmother? Since it is so far removed from what is expected, I think that some study of the whole set of events is called for. As a child reaches adolescence, they may begin to resent adult authority. This is natural, but it has to be contained. What was the provocation? Maybe a scolding given in the presence of friends or neighbours.

Talk to your daughter about her behaviour when she is in a good mood and tell her that she will be deprived of privileges if she continues to behave badly. But be consistent. Give her a set of rules that are reasonable, in your view, and make her sign a contract that she will observe them. Some children need an objective and visible method for rule keeping. Find out from her teachers if her school behaviour is acceptable. If she likes a particular aunt or teacher, that person can also help in validating the procedures you select. All this will work only if you express your affection to your daughter and make her realize that it is silly to be rude to those she loves. If this does not work, ask a psychologist to help you with the procedures in managing her.

118. How can I make my son realize that he is not a failure?

Q. My 10-year-old son believes that everyone is better than him in everything. He chooses friends that are dominating and aggressive. Though he is very active, yet he allows his friends to run over him, so to speak. For example, he allows them to win races or video games. He then believes that he is not good at these events. He enjoys playing various sports and has unlimited potential, but he holds himself back and beats himself up when he fails at the task. I took my son to a professional batting coach. In the first few weeks, I saw major improvement until he was struck out a couple of times. I encouraged him by saying that it is all right not to hit the ball every time or you'll get it next time. But now he is back to the old frame of mind and even the batting coach says its all in his head. After he strikes out, he holds his head down and cries behind his helmet. I believe I praise and encourage him in everything he does. But I don't push him to do things he doesn't want to do, unless it is his homework. I want to help but I don't know how. Any advice will be appreciated.

A. Too few facts have been presented for me to have a clear view. Apart from the mother, is there anyone else in the picture? Where is the father? Are there any siblings? It is clear that the boy wishes to punish himself for something he may have done or imagines to have done. One would need professional advice to get to the bottom of the masochistic tendency of the child.

Praise and encouragement are necessary and usually have a positive effect, but unqualified affection is also an essential part of the parenting dynamics. Maybe he could be allowed to have a pup as a pet and in bringing it up, learn something about growing up. That is only one suggestion. Maybe his class teacher could also be roped in as an ally in tackling this problem.

119. My son is bullied about his dark complexion, what should I do?

Q. My son is 10 years old. He is very intelligent and a sensitive child. Recently, I found a slight change in his behaviour. He gets angry too fast, without any reason. I thought it's due to the age factor but I came to know that it's due to his skin colour, which is very dark – not even wheatish. Both of us are of wheatish complexion. My son was fair when he was born, but he turned dark when olive oil was applied on him for massage. We are not so worried as he is a healthy and intelligent child. He reads a lot and knows the scientific reasons behind his colour. However, recently he has been bullied by a boy in his school bus about his skin colour. My son did not have the guts to tell me at first but after a lot of persuasion he told me that he has dreams in which he is able to take off his skin and get a fair skin. Should I see a psychiatrist to make him overcome this problem? Is there a skin treatment available for him?

A. Be happy that you have a bright and healthy child. Skin colour and pigmentation are not problems. However, I do see that the classmates he has in the school have made it a problem. I think you should talk to the head or principal of the school and have him talk about human values to the children. No trait, whether it is disability, skin colour or texture of hair should be considered a matter for discrimination. The school should take up this issue seriously and bring out the importance of friendship and good relationships.

Since your son does seem to be bothered enough about his skin to have dreams about fair skin, it would be a good idea to see a psychologist or psychiatrist, for at least a couple of sittings. Your role as parents in reassuring him that he is valued and loved by you should be emphasized. If there is an international school, which he can attend, he will see that people of all colours and sizes inhabit this world and no one is superior or inferior to another on the basis of appearance.

120. How to deal with a child who abuses and shouts while playing?

Q. My 12-year-old son is slightly hyperactive. He speaks in a loud tone, is very

fast at doing his tasks, fares well in studies but is obsessed with playing cricket. Sometimes while playing with his friends, he gets abusive but not violent. He has been hit by his friends badly and he reacts furiously screaming a volley of abuses but without hitting equally in return. He has a compassionate heart. He does play cricket with his friends often, yet he prefers to play cricket with me (his father), as he believes that I play better than many of his friends. How should we, as parents, deal with him?

A. Your son seems to be adjusting reasonably well to the demands of his environment. Cricket can be an interest, even a passion, and many people who were cricket-crazy as boys, have grown up to be successful adults.

However, shouting and being abusive can be very irritating to all who are present around him. His friends will not tolerate it, if it goes beyond limits. I think you will have to include other activities into his everyday schedule. He probably has the energy for more physical and mental activity.

It is heartening that he has a good relationship with his father. Use this for persuasion (to accept your values, for instance). An element of humour and playfulness could also be very useful to defuse tension, occasionally. As he will soon be a teenager, giving him some idea of the sexual development and physical changes in adolescence is also advised.

121. My daughter once got choked and is hence scared of eating, what do we do?

Q. My daughter is 11 years old. About a month back, while she was eating her meal, some food particles got stuck in her windpipe/throat. As a result, her throat got choked and after some efforts she was able to expel it out. But this turned out to be a terrifying experience for her. For the past 1 month she is scared of swallowing food and keeps chewing it and ultimately throws it out. She has lost about 2 kg due to this. She is taking only drinks or very soft food. I took her to a doctor. Since there was no medical problem diagnosed, the doctor could not suggest much. In fact, she has developed a fear psychosis. We have tried our best, doing everything from encouragement to extreme coercion, but she is not recovering from it. Can you please advise us on what should be done so that she resumes her normal eating habit?

A. Your daughter has developed a fear of choking on solid food after that traumatic experience. You can try to help her get over it by discussing her fear. She is old enough to see that she cannot starve any longer. Try to make her understand how she can overcome this fear, by taking gradual steps. Make sure she has enriched liquid foods such as chocolate milk or malt drinks, while she is in the process of getting over her problem. She can try with semi-solids, then move to small bites of solids. Encourage and praise her small steps to normalcy. In case the fear persists, you should consult a psychologist for assessment, counselling and intervention.

Sex education

122. How can I stop my child from surfing pornographic sites?

Q. My 12-year-old son is looking at pornographic pictures and sites on the internet, including gay sites. I have checked his history and found many such sites. Although we have talked about it before but I have found that he is still continuing with it. We have explained that curiosity is natural and have asked if he thinks he is gay but he insists he is just curious. At what point does this become an obsession and should one be concerned? He is a good kid, active in sports and a great student.

A. You are right in assuming that natural curiosity may impel children to search for porn sites on the computer.

Your son seems to have started early. The problem with viewing such sites is that it becomes a habit and never seems enough. I think you should instal a parental control software (like Net Nanny) that provides internet monitoring and website filtering, so that only certain sites will be available to your son. But tell him you are doing it and that it is in his interest. Be consistent and firm in the rules.

Tell him that he should now focus on studies, sports and having good friends who will like him and respect him.

Miscellaneous

123. Why is the child more attached to his uncle and aunt than his own parents?

Q. My nephew is 12 years old. He does not concentrate on his studies and is careless. His school teachers also say that he is not attentive in class. He had been taken care of by his grandmother till the age of 8. After his grandmother passed away, his aunt and uncle started taking care of his studies and the rest of the times he was with his parents. His aunt got married, and his uncle still somehow managed to take care of his studies. He lost his father this year and his mother is living away. The child is safe and happy with his uncle and aunt. He is so well-adjusted with them that he even wants to write his uncle's name instead of his father's. Now what to do with this child – how to handle him?

A. Every child needs emotional attachment with a parent figure, and this provides a sense of security and trust. The details provided in your query do not explain why the parents did not take care of the child. It is clear that many different relatives have looked after him. He may be suffering from a break in attachment after the grandmother's death. He also seems to be suffering from a sense of rejection by his parents. If the uncle is willing to accept the child, then there is no harm if the child is using his uncle's name. Perhaps it is the only name he trusts. He would benefit from proper psychological assessment and individual counselling.

Adolescents

- School issues
- Behaviour/habits

School issues

124. How can I make my nephew realize the importance of education?

Q. My sister's son is in grade 8. He is not interested in studying. He is more interested in computer hardware and says that he wants to discontinue his studies and go in the hardware field. He does not realize the importance of education and does not respect his parents at all. He is good at heart but is very adamant and always takes anyone's advice in the wrong way and my sister is worried. Please help us and suggest what we can do to make him understand the importance of education.

A. An 8th-grader is an adolescent and is probably going through a phase of identity confusion and formation. It is a phase when there can be a tendency to feel peer pressure and get distracted by several things. Parents are usually considered behind the times and out-of-date and they are not listened to. Also, children often say that they want to drop out of school and take care of puppies or make kites or whatever. They should not be taken literally 'as not being interested in education', but rather as a mild protest about school routines.

Rather than feeling disturbed at being disobeyed, make your nephew realize that education is necessary for becoming a computer hardware expert. Higher secondary schooling is essential to reach even a modest level of expertise later, or else he would remain a mere mechanic. He can also be introduced to persons working at different levels of computer hardware jobs, so that he can make up his mind what level he is aiming for. Help can be taken from his computer teachers at school.

125. How can I help my son to cope with higher studies?

Q. My son is a student of class XI, non-medical stream. Of late he has started worrying about not being able to keep up with the class. His confidence level has also reduced. He does not want to go to school and due to this guilt he feels that everyone is talking about him. I am afraid that he is suffering from anxiety neurosis. What is the best way to make him come out of this state of mind? Please advise.

A. Your child is undergoing a phase of severe anxiety crisis and lack of confidence. There is a sudden jump in difficulty level of courses from class X to XI. Children who have been high achievers at the junior levels often find this sudden jump difficult to cope with. He needs to get some professional help for his anxiety. Try and have him see a psychiatrist or psychologist.

As a parent you can take the following steps to help him.

- Get him regular professional counselling by the school counsellor.
- Listen to the child and acknowledge his fears rather than criticizing him.
- Arrange for tuition classes.
- Do not compare him with other children.
- Discuss the problem with his schoolteachers.
- Keep the option of changing the course open, even at this late stage.

126. I have exam phobia, what do I do?

Q. I have not appeared for the class 12 exams for the past 2 years due to phobia. I have dropped 2 years. Now, this is creating an inferiority complex. I feel like committing suicide. What should I do?

A. Passing a school exam is not the end of the world! I am sure you have some strong points. Try to focus and build on those. Remember that many great persons in history were not able to do well at school. It is also possible that you can do well, but are simply not appearing for the exam out of fear. The best option for you is to get professional help as soon as possible. Try to contact a school counsellor, or a psychologist or even a telephone helpline. It is possible to reduce or even remove the fear by proper counselling and psychotherapy. It is not your fault and many people are prone to such fears. Get emotional support from your parents or friends. (*See also* page 190)

127. Will my daughter's interest in movies and actors harm her studies?

Q. My elder daughter is 13 years old. She is good in studies. Both my husband and I are working and after school hours she and her younger sister stay alone at home till 6 p.m. My concern is that she is very fond of movies and serials. She doesn't want to see anything else. Nowadays she has started collecting pictures of Amrita Rao whom she likes a lot and is mad after her. Will this harm her studies? How can I tackle her? Also, she has a habit of sleeping till 9 a.m. on holidays. I shout at her for these things, which I know is not good. How can I control myself? I realize that these are teenage fads but still I want some satisfactory answer from you.

A. You are right in understanding that your daughter is passing through adolescence, which can be a period of stress. Getting up late, interest in movies and television, hero-worshipping, etc. are typical of this stage. You admit that she is good in studies, which means that she is able to balance her teenage interests with academic achievement. What is wrong with sleeping late on a holiday? Relax your rules a little and things may settle down. Try to be good role models yourselves and be consistent in disciplining. Use a mixture of firm discipline, warmth and stability of family environment.

128. How do I improve my concentration in studies?

Q. I feel restless as exams approach. I do not feel comfortable while studying. I am a retentive person and usually get bored even when I hold a book in my hand. Please give an effective solution so that I can concentrate more on my studies.

A. The problems faced by you are not uncommon, but they can prove to be a hindrance in effective study. Restlessness during studying could be a sign of anxiety and fatigue, but it could also be due to wrong posture, lack of interest, or presence of distraction in the environment. Since you also mention boredom, it is possible that you need to make some changes in your study environment and habits. Try the following suggestions.

- Make a realistic study schedule, incorporating sufficient rest periods.
- Alternate easy with difficult subjects, boring with interesting ones.
- Choose a specific place to study, which should be free of distractions such as telephone and television.

- Use a table and chair while studying and ensure good posture and good lighting.
- If you are not able to concentrate, take a break and then come back refreshed.
- Plan short-term targets for yourself.
- Reward yourself for successful study periods.

(*See also* page 190)

129. Why is my son using bad words in school?

Q. My 13-year-old son has been using bad words in school. In a monthly test held recently, instead of writing the answer to the question, he wrote all bad words related to anal sex. What should I do in such a situation? The principal called my wife and me and threatened to suspend the child from school, if not expel him. Please advise.

A. The first thing to do is to talk to your son and ask him why he wishes to use words related to anal sex. If you are open and mature about it, he may discontinue his use of such words. You should also explain to him that his sexual organs are growing and related aspects of sexuality are also developing. It is normal for boys at this age to be thinking of their body, more than ever before. But, it is certainly not common to write sexual words in a test! He should also be advised to see a psychologist or a school counsellor, who will help him to put his bodily impulses in the context of early adolescence.

Boys of his age may use bad words (which may not be really bad, but only presented at the wrong time and improper context, with the intention of shocking others). At other times, the intention is to show-off. These words could also be used to express anger or aggression. You and his mother should be concerned about your son's behaviour, but handle it gently and with some humour. Get professional help. Make a request to the school to let him continue there, while you are actively addressing the issues related to the boy's sex education and to the handling of his anger. (*See also* pages 50, 101)

Behaviour/habits

130. How can I help my daughter give up the habit of chatting on the net?

Q. My 15-year-old daughter seems unable to give up her habit of chatting on the net with her friends despite repeated reasoning by me. I want her to concentrate more on her studies, and cut down on telephone expenses. I have explained to her that if we can cut down on wasteful expenses, I will have more money to buy some of the things she wants. She is otherwise intelligent and reasonable but she lapses into the chatting habit all the time. Should I detach the modem, which will effectively prevent her from connecting to the net? She seems to get depressed when she is unable to chat. Also, she enjoys long conversations on the phone. How should I tackle this problem? What should I do if she gets depressed if I stop the chatting altogether? She is normally of a cheerful disposition and I don't want her to get grumpy and unhappy especially in view of her impending board exams next year?

A. I think your daughter is old enough to realize that she has to plan her time to include lessons, games and friends. Help her to make a detailed daily timetable and see how much of her time is spent in chatting on the net. Explaining only in terms of how the money (spent on calls) can be spent better is obviously not having the needed impact.

She must give you an undertaking that she will not spend more than 50–60 minutes a day on the net, chatting with friends. If she is not amenable to the suggestion, you will have to shift the computer to a central room, where there will not be much privacy for her. If this is not possible, you will have to say that she is on trust to keep to the time limit.

When the next telephone bill comes and reflects her long chatting hours on the chat-line, tell her that she must be prepared to have the modem cut off. Of course, she will sulk a bit, but I can't imagine that it will do a great deal of harm. Children have different levels of sensitivity and you will be the best judge of how strict you can be. Explain to her that her performance in the board exams will practically open or shut doors for all future decisions. She should do as well as she can, without feeling over-pressured. Connect her present activities to her hopes for the future. She will probably tell you that she is discussing her homework with her classmates! Be firm in your rules for her, but have a touch of gentleness and a bit of humour in your interaction. If you can get her father or others in the family also to support your views, it would have a better impact. Her good marks in term exams etc. will become a reward for hard work. But she has to feel motivated herself. You can only help it along. She is at the difficult age of 15. It will be much better in a year from now.

131. Why does my son treat his sister as a rival?

Q. I have a 16-year-old son. His main complaint is that we don't give him much time and we are more affectionate towards his sister who is 10 years old. He gives the same reason for his non-performance in the exams and demands that we help him study as we help his sister (class VI). He is a good student, we know and have told him that we are confident that he can perform still better. Is it true that due to this perception his grades might go down? What should be done to get him out of this wrong perception? Has he lost his self-esteem? His sister gets much better grades than him, participates in elocution, dance and drama. He also participates in elocution and drama and is the preferred speaker in his school. He is very helpful, responsible, reads a lot of news, magazines and has a good general knowledge. How do we help him?

A. You are lucky to have two high-performing children! Start with counting your blessings!

Sibling rivalry or the feeling of competition between two children in the same family is very common. You have to dispel the child's feeling of bias against him or bias in favour of his sister. Once in a while, you can also sit with him while he is studying, chatting in between and doing your own work, so that he gets a feeling of companionship. Because a child is bright and talented, we tend to treat him as a grown up. A 16-year-old also needs an occasional cuddle and a joke shared with him.

The very fact that you say that his sister gets much better grades than him indicates the constant comparison. It is difficult, but you must feel and be able to indicate that each child is valuable and loved, irrespective of school performance. After a couple of times of your helping him in his studies, he will want to be free to do his own work. Self-esteem is not a lost-and-found object. It is built up over a period of time, through several interactions with parents and others. Instead of pushing him to do better, tell him if he does well enough to get the course he wants, you will be satisfied. As soon as the pressure of parental expectations is off, he will start doing his best. Indulge him a little, instead of being stern. It seems he wants that assurance.

132. How can I cope with the comparison made by my parents?

Q. I am always being tortured at home and my parents constantly compare me with my brother. They scold me for no mistake of mine, as I am not as good at studies as him. I am very worried about this and get severe headaches at times. I don't smoke or drink alcohol. Please advise.

A. You seem to have developed a sense of inadequacy and frustration at being compared and scolded. Adolescence and young adulthood can be especially difficult times. Remember that all individuals are different. Learn to identify your own strong points and build on them. Stop focusing on your weaknesses. You cannot change others but you can change the way you think and react. Rather than thinking that you are being tortured, try to think that your parents want your improvement and welfare. Try to communicate with your parents. Express your anguish and need for love and approval without blaming them or being rude. Talk to a friend to share your feelings. Better still, learn stress management and take professional help from a qualified psychologist or counsellor.

133. My adolescent son has a habit of pulling his hair, what should I do?

Q. My son, who is 14 years old, has a habit of pulling his hair and meddling with it, especially, while studying and eating his food. I am afraid that this habit might interfere with his studies. So please help me.

A. Adolescents are very sensitive and too much interference in their personal habits is not desirable. It may even rebound and make the child rebellious. Try to ignore the behaviour and make a constructive suggestion when he is in a receptive mood. Take care not to repeat yourself or be derogatory. Behaviour of this sort may be transitory and pass off soon. Why do you connect everything to studies? Give some importance to his emotional and social development too.

134. How can I help my adolescent son make friends?

Q. My son is 14 years old. His problem is that he does not have friends. He always has the fear that nobody would talk to him and none of his friends would listen to him. Please tell me how can I help him develop a personality so that he can get along well with people and make good friends.

A. Your son is going through the period of adolescence which can be often stressful. Identity crisis and peer acceptance are very important issues at this age. Generally, children at this age feel inadequate and shy. As a parent you can help by:

- Not making him conscious of his lack of friends or lack of social skills. Do not label your child, as it will reduce his self-confidence. Do not compare or criticize him and do not force him to do anything. If you are relaxed, he will relax and be natural too.
- Praising his positive points to build his self-esteem. Every person does have some strengths. Identify and encourage them.
- Letting him join a club or a sports group where he can learn social skills and get opportunity to meet people and make friends.

135. How should I handle my daughter having a boyfriend?

Q. How should I handle my adopted daughter who is 17 years old? I was separated when she was 9 years old. I found that she has a boyfriend when she was in 1st year, high school. I gave her an ultimatum that if she continues with that kind of attitude, she'll have to stop going to school. But her relationship didn't stop and now she's about to enroll in college. I am having second thoughts about enrolling her. I think I should stop her schooling to give her a lesson. What is the best way to handle this situation?

A. First and foremost, you will have to think about the child as your daughter, not as your adopted daughter. Many parents who adopt seem to come upon some problems when the child reaches adolescence, because at the back of their mind, they think some genetic factors are manifesting. Actually, the very same problems are faced by biological parents. You certainly should not deny her an education as a punishment for having a boy as a friend. What lesson will you teach her? With nothing to do and a lot of resentment at having her movements curbed, she is likely to have more serious problems.

Talk to her about herself, her growing up and the responsibilities she has towards her own future. All parents have to do this. Do not surrender your responsibility with a militaristic ultimatum! Times have changed since we were at this age, whether we like it or not! Youngsters have a mind of their own and will only accept what they consider reasonable. But they need your affection, firmness and consistency. They need discussions to clarify their confusions. An authoritarian approach, with rule-quoting alone, will not help the situation. At the same time, you have to protect her from drugs and promiscuity, and have patience in doing so. If you handle this sensitive period well, you will have a daughter and friend for life. Talk to a counsellor or psychologist, if you need information on methods of handling the situation.

Appendix

I. Speech disorders
II. Learning issues
III. Television viewing
IV. Adolescent health
V. Coping with exams
VI. Resources

Speech disorders*

Q. Are children born with speech disorders or do they develop over time?

A. The reorganization of speech disorder is possible only when one has reached the stage of language acquisition skills. As the child grows you would accept certain sequential development in language skills. If the child has not developed these language skills during that period of time then we would be able to uncover them.

Q. At what age do children start speaking sentences?

A. At the age of one, the child speaks at least two words with meaning. There would be mamma, papa at least. At two years, they start putting two words together. They start understanding speech much earlier than talking and if there is a problem with understanding, then there could be a problem. But the child develops problems with speaking much later; it is then that we realize that it is a case of speech disorder.

Q. What are speech disorders? If a child babbles and then picks on words, is that a disorder? Or Is speaking late a disorder?

A. Speech disorders are of various types. There are certain disorders which occur due to the way you speak, due to problem in the voice, because of fluency and due to articulation. However, there are other disorders – some are associated with understanding language, receptive language disorder; and some are associated with speaking, expressive language disorder. These are clubbed together as speech and language disorders in children.

---

* Based on the transcript of a live Q&A programme telecast on NDTV 24X7

Whenever we talk about speech disorders, we look at four major factors. First, how clear is the speech? Second is the fluency aspect. Is the speech flowing smoothly, word after word or is the child hesitating? Other disorders are voice problems, where the child's voice is not free and normal. The loudness angle; when there is hearing loss and the child can't hear properly then he tends to talk loudly. When there is delayed and inadequate development of language, it is also classified as a speech disorder.

Q. If the problem is detected early, then will the treatment be quicker and more effective?

A. Yes, certainly; where hearing loss is concerned, a little bit of intervention does help. But generally, speech disorders become apparent around the age of 1-and-a-half years or later, because that is when the child starts using sentences. Then we try to see if an intervention is necessary, because as normal children go through speech development there is a little hiccup along the way and we don't classify that as a speech disorder. If after two years the issue inhibits the child's socialization or expression, we try to look at factors, which can be alleviated and help the child towards normal development.

Q. My son is 3 years old. He started doing everything late. He has still not started speaking, what should we do at this stage?

A.The parents should take him for a complete developmental evaluation, looking at all areas of development not only in language but other areas as well to see where the cause lies.

Q. My 18-year-old brother is studying engineering. He is good at technical things but when it comes to speech, he lacks some skills and his voice is not good. He reads very well but is not able to speak properly. Please advise.

A. It seems he is not able to maintain fluency. It is a problem of stammering and stuttering, where fluency is not maintained, especially in a stressful situation. When he is alone and comfortable, he is able to speak well. But whenever he is under stress, the speech gets disturbed. Fluency disorder can be alleviated. Generally, in this disorder, there is no problem while singing or recitation, but when it comes to spontaneous speech under pressure, he needs to learn how to clear up his innate expression and get the obstacle that interferes his fluency out of the way.

Q. **My younger son has a speech problem. He is not very clear and he stammers since birth. My elder son also had the same problem, but he overcame it. Can I do something to improve his speech?**

A. Sometimes, unclear speech and dis-fluency go hand in hand. In your child's case, the fact that elder brother had this issue might have been responsible for the younger one to also pick up this manner of talking. We must work towards finding out why the child is unclear, because many times if the child is not clear then the response he gets from his teachers can put speech under stress and as a result stuttering or stammering might develop. When we talk about unclear speech, we look at the movements of the tongue because clarity is dependent on the precise movement of the tongue. Tongue is a muscle; if it is used in a correct manner then the speech is clear. The movement of the tongue is sometimes hindered by a condition called a tongue-tie, where the ligament under the tongue is short and it doesn't facilitate the movement of the tongue especially in sounds, where it needs lingual elevation that means the tongue has to go up. If intervention is done at an early stage, the results are good and there is a little optimism in the prognosis. Since the elder brother had the same issue and he got over it, it augurs well for the younger brother also.

Q. **What are the causes for speech disorders? Are they genetic and can they be controlled beforehand?**

A. There are many causes of speech and language disorders. The most important thing we should keep in mind when there is delayed speech and language is whether the child's hearing is normal or not. Hearing impairment becomes a very important cause when somebody has a speech and language problem.

Q. **If someone speaks fast without punctuations or commas and he is aware that he speaks fast, is that a disorder?**

A. Certainly, a person who speaks fast does not convey his ideas in a pleasant and attractive manner. Speaking very fast is called cluttering. This is dependent upon the person's neurological makeup because all of us have a timer inside our body. He will have to regularly practice a slower rate of talking and for that he will have to take the help of an external device, which helps and gives him clues about when to talk.

When a person talks fast, he becomes breathless because whenever we talk, we exhale air and air is the power for speech. If I talk and don't stop in the middle, my lungs don't refill air. He will have to start practicing a slower and a more clear way of talking and for that he will have to talk with his mouth a little more open. When people clutter their sounds, they do not open their mouth adequately, so there is that microsecond speeding up of speech. He would benefit by practicing how to talk with his mouth open in private where he will be more comfortable. It will add clarity to the speech. It will reduce the time and will enhance vocal projection, which will make his speech clear over the phone.

Q. Are speech disorders due to some deficiency?

A. Deficiencies do not cause speech and language problems.

Learning issues*

Q. What are the learning issues in children?

A. Many children are smart and have lots of abilities in many areas, but they have difficulties in school due to the way their brains are wired. They are different from other individuals in their learning. Some children may have difficulty in mathematics because they have a particular memory problem. Others, though smart, may have trouble in reading. This may be due to their inability to deal with some aspects of language such as the sounds or to figure out complicated sentences. These children often appear lazy or people say that they are poorly motivated. They have an unusual pattern of brain wiring which causes this difficulty.

Q. Parents often get hysterical about their child not doing well in school. Or sometimes they are laid back. Can parents recognize these problems in their children?

A. Parents generally show three kinds of reactions. Some parents get too upset about it and others just ignore it. But it is best to recognize the problem and keep a good eye on it rather than getting nervous about it. If your child is struggling with reading or has trouble concentrating in school; if he is disorganized or seems to have a trouble in a particular area, for example he might not be able to spell or is a child who sounds good when he talks but is poor on paper; these could be typical signs of child who has some underlying dysfunction that is affecting his learning.

* Based on the transcript of a live Q&A programme telecast on NDTV 24X7

Q. It is often seen in siblings that one child is faster, understands quicker and is able to grasp things and retain them while the other is not. What in the brain triggers this condition?

A. It is something in the way a particular child's brain is set so that one child may have no difficulty in processing information quickly but the other may take longer to do so. But that same child who takes too long to process information may be wonderful in doing things with his hands which his sister or brother can't. He may be much more creative. Every child has a profile of strengths and weaknesses in memory, in language, in concentration and in the ability to reason or solve problems.

Q. Who can identify this problem, can parents do it or do they have to see an expert?

A. Parents need to be the first one to suspect that their child has trouble expressing himself or he is doing poorly in tests or he is having a lot of problem with mathematics or reading too slowly. Sometimes the child develops behavioural problems because he is embarrassed and humiliated due to his learning difficulties. Even a behaviour problem can be a sign of learning problem. Once the parents suspect that there is a problem, they often need help from an expert who can evaluate the child, who can figure out what his strengths and weaknesses are, who can pinpoint what is getting in the way when the child tries to learn maths or tries to write. He has to evaluate whether it is a memory problem, a language problem, a trouble in visualizing things or a motor problem. We need an expert to find out where the breakdown is occurring and then we can do something about it.

Q. Are these problems very common in our country? How many parents go to a specialist in this regard?

A. These problems are as common in our country as they would be in the western world, but the only thing is that parents often misdiagnose and misunderstand such problems to be signs of laziness, not wanting to work enough and punitive action is taken. Parents or teachers deal with it in a very nasty way either through punishment, by labeling the child as weak or slow and it becomes a cyclic pattern. As behavioural problems can result from these learning differences, the vice versa is also true, as sometimes behavioural problems or emotional blocks could be the root of learning differences.

Q. **In our country most schools are supposed to have a counsellor. In case the counsellors are not there, then where should the parents take the child to identify the problem and to work upon it?**

A. You are right; it is mandatory to have a counsellor in every school today. It's another matter how good is the counsellor's work, but at least there is one. The first person to recognize and identify these issues should be the teacher and the parents and such issues should be directed to the school counsellor. Besides that you can go to a child specialist, clinical psychologist or paediatrician who will refer you to the right person.

Q. **How do you tell a person that he should follow a certain pattern to maximize his concentration level?**

A. First of all, someone who is having trouble in concentrating needs to find out the best time of the day to concentrate. He might find that he is a night person or a morning person. He needs to give himself plenty of breaks when he works. Sometimes listening to music while working makes a difference. So he has to experiment on what works on his attention and how can he maximize his power of concentration.

Q. **How can we identify the skills of my 2-year-old girl?**

A. Two years is too early an age. At this age there are definitely some interests and some attitudes which can be identified but there is no hard and fast rule and diagnostic tools are not sophisticated enough. We can see whether the child has reached certain developmental milestones and try to identify certain strengths and encourage those. In India, at the age of 2 years, parents send their children to preschool and the child is taught how to read and write and the child develops a sense of failure, inadequacy and it can carry on later in life. The child may feel there is too much pressure in school and learning can be very unpleasant.

Q. **Are children born with learning dysfunctions or do they arise later in life?**

A. Many children are born with a tendency to have learning problems. It is unclear whether that tendency would become a serious problem or remain a mild problem. But a lot of it is in the genes or something that happens during pregnancy – it is part of the wiring of the child. We have to realize that and be careful. It is inhuman to punish, disgrace or embarrass a child for something, which is not his fault. Often these learning problems result in accusing the child of being lazy or poorly motivated and the child is kept back in a grade and brutalized in school.

Q. Where do you think we lag behind in our country and what should be done so that we can bring out the best in the children who are suffering from this problem?

A. We, Indians, respect learning issues. Unfortunately, we are rote learners and there is too much emphasis on examinations, on rote learning, on theory and less emphasis on understanding – project work and demonstrations. We should encourage children to understand and develop motivation and interest in the subject rather than just learning like a parrot.

Television viewing*

Q. Is television viewing harmful?

A. The harms of television viewing are that the child loses out quality time of parent interaction, for studies, for play, for physical activity and for good quality eating. Direct consequences of TV viewing include a lot of visual stimulation, which could be in terms of vision, contact or reading. TV provides advance system of stimulation to the brain, so it is the visual stimulus that overwhelms all other stimulation very early in life, which is not conducive for good brain development. There are some studies which say that a lot of television viewing lead to problems such as hyperactivity, attention deficit disorders and even may contribute to learning difficulties. Television viewing also has other problems. For example, if you are not watching from a good distance, it could have a direct effect on vision. It could precipitate fits in patients who are otherwise predisposed.

Q. What are the psychological impacts of TV? Is it related to the kind of programme a child watches?

A. Definitely, whatever you present to the child is going to have an impact. If you present meaningless loud noise to a very young child, it is going to be harmful. A lot of people seem to treat television viewing as a babysitting exercise – just put the child in front of the television and hope the baby will be quiet. That is the worst thing to do because babies like to have silence; they like sounds that can be understood and vision that can be comprehended.

* Based on the transcript of a live Q&A programme telecast on NDTV 24X7

Q. **What is the role of parents between the TV and the child?**

A. Parents have a very important role because the habit of television viewing stems down from the parents. Parents should focus on what should be watched and when it should be watched. Even if a programme is exceptionally good and instructive, it is not good if it is watched all day. A child needs multiple stimulations all through the day, so it's a question of the quantum and the time. If it is time for the child to do his homework or play in the garden, then it is not ideal for him to watch television. All programmes that are for adults are not necessarily suited for children. Something that stimulates the child and provides information in a manner that is conducive for the development is fine. But information that is redundant to the child's development, non-instructive, non-informative and that does not create a happy situation for the child is not suitable for his viewing. It's not necessary that all programme that are watched by adults need to be watched by the family together. The parents should select the programmes to see what is suitable depending on the age and development of the child. There is no doubt that TV is a powerful medium of instruction and entertainment to the child but you need to moderate what they watch.

Q. **Can cartoon watching stimulate the thinking of a young child?**

A. We have very little choice as compared to other countries. We have not paid enough attention to television for children. There is even a children's film society, which has so many films but these are never telecast at a time when children can view it on television. We need more children-friendly programmes; some exists but are not enough.

Q. **How does television viewing affect the eyes?**

A. The effects on the eyes are multifold. When you watch TV from a very close distance without adequate lighting, it can have a direct effect on the eyes. There are certain frequencies and geometric patterns that influence the eye in a detrimental manner. Prolonged watching from very close distance can strain your eye muscles.

Q. **Is colour television worse than black and white television?**

A. In terms of stimulation to produce photosensitive epilepsy, black and white was worse. Colour TV is not worse than black and white TV, but what is important is that there are certain children who are predisposed by these frequencies to develop certain electrical discharges in the brain, which are not conducive for them.

Q. Should we curtail our children from watching steamy videos on TV?

A. These videos are not at all meant for children to watch. There are other kinds of music that a child can learn. There are so many things in our own traditional music that can be fun for children.

Q. How do you discourage a child from watching excessive TV?

A. One would have to sit down with the child and have a serious discussion and listen to the child also. One has to tell them that these are the things they have to do, make a timetable for them. Tell the child how much time is to be spent in front of the television. Make your child understand that excessive TV viewing is meaningless. Parents should also provide some other interesting things that the child can do.

Q. What kind of programmes can children watch? My 3-year-old son only watches cartoon network, I don't know how to tell him to stop. What should be the duration of TV viewing?

A. Cartoon network is very stereotypic. It's not instructive and creative, does not have a variety of stimulation and educational experience. It is not the greatest channel for children. A good channel for children would be the one that shows good old stories enacted very well.

Q. My 2-and-a-half-year-old son is interested in watching TV ads; otherwise, he is generally uninterested. He becomes very aggressive. Is the TV affecting him?

A. Excessive television viewing results in a number of behaviour problems. Being irritable and aggressive could be one of them. We should avoid seeing very stimulating ads that display a lot of aggression. A lot of times, physical activity takes away aggression from the child's behaviour. If a child goes and plays a game of football or cricket with other children in that extra time, it may be far more meaningful.

Q. **For how long should a child be allowed to watch television?**

A. Ideally, it should be 30–40 minutes a day. More than 40 minutes of TV viewing is not at all required for 12–13-year olds. For a very young child, the duration should be even less.

Q. **Is watching TV and obesity related to each other?**

A. When you sit and watch television, most of the time you eat junk food without any regular meal and you don't have any interaction with others. In addition, it takes away a lot of physical activity time. Somehow the above two run in the families where children are permitted to watch a lot of television and have a lot of freedom to eat anything they like. The ads of junk food on TV also promote this.

Q. **From how much distance should one watch television?**

A. The normal TV watching distance should be about 3 and a half metres and should generally be in a straight line to that of the television. The lights should preferably be behind the television.

Q. **At what age is a child mature enough to take the decision on what to watch?**

A. At 18 years of age, but only with sensible parental guidance.

Adolescent health*

Q. What is the adolescent age period in a child?

A. By the WHO definition, the age 10–19 years is called an adolescent period.

Q. What is it that happens to children in this age group?

A. Many changes are occurring in the body of an adolescent. They are about to start with puberty and this makes the girls and boys very conscious. They suddenly do not have the same self-esteem as they may have had before. It is often observed that confident children suddenly become withdrawn, very conscious because they can't cope up with their body image, and they want to be either thin or fat or whatever they are not.

Q. Children do not go through the physical changes at the same time. How do you explain to a child that it is all right if his physical changes are not the same as everybody else's.

A. This is a very important point. We call them early bloomers or late bloomers. If in a class where all the children are feeling a certain body pattern and one boy does not develop a moustache, or one girl does not get her breast changes, they feel very conscious and are ridiculed. As parents and doctors, we have to make teenagers aware that it is all right to get your puberty a year later or a year earlier. This is part of a normal process.

* Based on the transcript of a live Q&A programme telecast on NDTV 24X7

Q. Other than body changes, is there any other way in which teenagers feel inadequate?

A. The best thing for them is to have an open communication channel with their parents, because they are not only going through their body changes; they are also going through emotional changes. They are no longer kids, but are not adults either. They also have physical and mental attraction to the opposite sex, and have a lot of confusing things going through their minds. This leads to lack of self-confidence. Parents can explain that all this is normal.

Q. At this age many teenagers want to be like all the top models in the country, which causes a lot of problems such as anorexia etc. How can parents help?

A. The parents should help children recognize the right diet, the right nutrition and the right body image. What the children see on the TV may not be necessarily healthy. Girls may be prone to an eating disorder such as anorexia nervosa in which they stop eating because they are afraid to put on weight.

Q. Is there any right or wrong way of communicating with the child?

A. Actually, it's a communication between two individuals, so there is nothing right or wrong but what is best for the child. One understands through experience that if I talk to my child in a certain way, he responds, and is not rebellious, he is not rude and is cooperative. One general observation is that most adolescents get very upset if they are ridiculed.

Q. Do you think that comparing your child with other children will make them more rebellious?

A. This is the worst thing to do to an adolescent. If you compare an adolescent with your neighbour's child or other siblings, you really create a lot of problems for this child. Each child is a unique individual and, therefore, you have to handle them as individuals.

Q. **When should you start giving the adolescent freedom or decision-making powers?**

A. Yes, one should start giving at least some amount of freedom to them. You should involve them in the decision-making. For example, if you say that you have to watch TV only for 1 hour and you have to study for 4 hours, let the teenager decide at what time that 1 hour should be. We cannot force them to study at a particular time.

Q. **I am 15 years old and I have lots of hair on my body, but these days I see actors who do not have a single hair on their body. I get an inferiority complex when I wear my shorts. What should I do?**

A. First thing is that, in the past, men liked to have hair on the body. It was considered manly and most women liked it, but nowadays men also remove their hair. If you are feeling so conscious about it, there are various ways by which hair can be removed. Your sister or your mother can help you or you can go to a doctor, but it is all right to have hair on the body, don't feel conscious about it, otherwise, you will develop more problems.

Q. **How should parents handle sexual curiosity in adolescents?**

A. This is a very, very important question and a majority of children are not comfortable with their sexuality because their parents have not discussed sexuality with them. Parents are often very embarrassed when their adolescent openly asks them questions related to sex. Either they tell them to shut up or they try to avoid the question by saying something else. But please remember, if as parents you do not satisfy the curiosity of your teenager, he will definitely find other sources to satisfy this curiosity and this may lead to procuring wrong information from the internet, from friends or it may be from somebody else. Therefore, if your adolescent asks questions about sex, please be open and forthright, and discuss the issue with them.

You can take your child to a doctor. You can also find somebody in your family who can answer. You can also take them to school but don't try to avoid or don't try to ridicule or make them ashamed that they have asked you this question.

Q. **My son is 14 years old. He's not able to concentrate on his studies and his eating habits are poor. What should I do?**

A. I think, first of all you need to have a heart-to-heart talk with your son. May be he is having some problems in his school or with his friends. Something is definitely bothering him, which is creating all these behavioural changes. Once you find out what the problem is, you can help him to deal with it. You will find that his behaviour will come back to normal.

Q. **Drugs are a major problem in schools nowadays and teenagers catch on to them very easily. How can parents keep them away from drugs?**

A. Again, in families where you have excellent communication between the parents and the children, there will be less drug abuse and the children will do much better. But the important point is that the parents should make an effort to understand what are drugs and their bad effects. How to pick up the signs that your child is using drugs? Generally, children whose parents are divorced or are always out of the house, children who get tremendous amount of pocket money and do not have any parental supervision are the ones to use drugs. And of course, you must know what sort of company your child is keeping. If the friends are experimenting with drugs, it is likely that your child is going to experiment with drug too.

Coping with exams*

Q. Is there a correct time for children to study, e.g. in the morning or at night?

A. Some children like to study in the morning and others at night. Some children can study very well in the night when everybody else is sleeping, but there could be others who wake up early morning to do their best. So parents should let the children draft their own timings for studies.

Q. Are taking breaks in between studying important and for how long should these breaks be?

A. Again, it depends on the individual child. There may be a child who can study non-stop for 2 hours and then take a break or a child who will be distracted within an hour. The parent and child should understand when the break is required and they should monitor adequate number of breaks. It is very important to keep taking breaks because if your mind gets tired, you may sit at the table for long hours looking at the books and end up grasping nothing.

Q. Is there a correct diet that children should follow to be more attentive?

A. It is very important to have a well-balanced diet because a good healthy diet of vegetables, fibre and fruits, helps the mind to stay alert whereas heavy junk food such as pizza etc. slows down the brain. So, after a very heavy meal, especially junk food, the brain doesn't function optimally. Secondly, if you keep taking stimulants in the diet, e.g. tea,

* Based on the transcript of a live Q&A programme telecast on NDTV 24X7

coffee, chocolates, it does stimulate you to some extent but only to fatigue you later.

Q. **Is it a good idea to continue tuitions during exams?**

A. This depends on the nature of the tutor. If the tutor is going to help the child revise everything in a manner that the child will not be able to do himself or herself, then it may be helpful. But I think we cannot really fix any rules for all children. There are so many different types of kids, with different habits, that it is important we respect their individuality.

Q. **How can a teacher in school make the children comfortable with what they are studying?**

A. Whether it is the teacher or the parent, I think everyone has to understand that a child ought to work to his individual capacity and too much of pushing at the last minute will not help. The teacher's role is very important from the beginning of the term till the end, but more specifically, at the end of the term or when the exams are going to begin.

Q. **There are instances of children getting depressed nowadays, especially when exams are closer. What can be done about this?**

A. Examination time is a period of anxiety and nervousness for the child. This is a period when parents and teachers also get worried about their child's performance. This happens because so far in our country, we have one 3-hour examination to decide the fate of the child. To face these 3 hours confidently, regular studies are required along with periodic assessment.

Q. **My daughter gets nervous before the exams. Please help.**

A. Everybody gets nervous before the exams and to tackle it at that time, as an emergency, does not work. What parents should do from the very beginning is to help the child calm down and follow some relaxation exercises. This can be done in the form of meditation or body stretching exercises. If you know how to make your mind tranquil from the beginning, it helps when the exam time approaches. But what happens is that most parents do not make any efforts throughout the year and when exams approach and the children are nervous, they want to suddenly learn to calm them, which is not easy.

Q. Do you think that nowadays sports and physical activity have become less and children rather sit on the computer or go for tuitions. Does this affect their mindset?

A. Majority of children and parents feel that taking part in any sort of physical activity, especially during class 12 is a waste of time. Exercise is not only important for the body to be functional but it has been shown that exercise releases good hormones called endorphins that relax the body and the mind. I would, therefore, like to ask all parents to allow their children to have at least half an hour of some physical exercise which is as important as studying. It will not waste their time but rather help them perform much better.

Q. Since examination time is a time when both parents and children are very nervous, is it helpful if parents accompany their kids to the examination centre?

A. I think it is perfectly all right for parents to accompany their children because it is the comfort level that matters and most children want the parents to be around them. There are, however, some students who feel very embarrassed or some parents have no time for their children.

We should also ask the child because there are some children who do want their parents with them while there are some who don't want their parents to accompany them, especially the adolescent boys who feel very independent. Let the child decide whether they want their parents to accompany them or not.

Q. Even when I am well prepared before the exams, I forget everything when I am revising the night before the exam and I have to prepare all over again. What shall I do?

A. There is an element of anxiety in the mind of every student. He thinks he has forgotten everything, but probably when he reaches the examination hall he realizes that he knows everything. It is an expression of disturbance and nervousness and it is natural.

Another reason is that most students feel that they should revise the entire course all over again the night before the exam. This is just not possible. So, children should relax the night before the exam and just go over the important points for revision. They cannot complete the whole course in one night.

Q. Can you give us a few tips on answering difficult questions?

A. To overcome the level of difficulty in answering the questions, read the question paper very carefully and then for a moment, stress on your mind and note down mentally what could be the answer, but don't immediately start writing. If you feel that you do not know the answer immediately or your recall memory is failing you, then leave a little space for that answer and go ahead. After you have done all the ones that seem easy, come back to the difficult question and if you have really studied the syllabus thoroughly, the answer will definitely come back to you.

Q. Parents are being blamed to be putting a lot of pressure on their children by comparing them to neighbours' children or a friend's child. What do you say?

A. Parents need to realize that they cannot have unrealistic expectations. They should be aware of what their child is capable of getting - 95% or 60%, and then can always help him and support him to get a little more. But you can't expect the 60 percenter to score 95% only because you are nagging or pushing him. So, what I feel is that parents should be a solid rock behind their children, giving them unconditional love and helping them to realize their best potential but not to have unrealistic expectations.

Q. I am a final-year literature student; the main problem with me is that I haven't studied the whole year, and now it's 4 days before the exam and I don't feel like studying. Is there any way of answering the papers in a much more impressive way to score higher marks? Is it important to go through the previous year question papers?

A. Yes, it is very important to go through the question papers of at least 5 previous years; if the books, pattern, or the syllabus has not changed. Since you have not studied throughout the year and you want some very quick solution or magical touch for success in the examination, you should go to your teacher and she should be able to give you some important tips. Never give up hope because examination is a great chance. Some people who work very, very hard don't show up with flying colours as compared to those who have just done last-minute preparation.

Q. How does an examiner who checks the answer papers recognize a good answer?

A. These days, the CBSE has given very clear-cut instructions for evaluating an answer. The best way to make your answer attractive is to write in a good handwriting and underline main parts of the answer. Also, it is imperative that the students understand the importance of word limit.

Q. I am a single parent. All I do is talk to my child and find out how he is preparing and how he has done, but I still feel inadequate. What shall I do?

A. There is no need to feel inadequate. A single parent may not be as well as both parents, but still you can do everything that is needed for the child. You should establish a good line of communication with your child. Though the child will miss the other parent, he will still be happy with you. Do not lose confidence in yourself. Be frank with your child and the child will open up to you too. I think, counselling is very important for both the child and the single parent to cope up with this inadequate feeling - why the other parent has left them? It is important to understand this, otherwise, the unhappiness can have a tremendous affect on the child's studies. Once the child understands the dynamics, he will feel much more secure and will do much better.

Q. When I go to the examination room, I start feeling very nervous and I nearly forget all that I have revised. What should I do?

A. This is actually an anxiety syndrome, and there are various methods of dealing with this anxiety such as meditation, relaxation exercises, calming the mind, etc. If the anxiety syndrome is very severe, it is better to take a doctor's help so that he can provide the right guidance.

Q. Do you think discussing the question paper after an exam is important?

A. Yes, of course, its natural for a student to want to know how he has done in the examination. But you should choose the person with whom you are discussing the paper. He should not discourage you or make you feel that you have done badly.

Q. Children tend to get depressed before the exams and probably get into suicidal thoughts. Is there any way of identifying such students?

A. It is very important for parents as well as siblings to understand that a particular child is suffering from depression. Most children who are likely to commit suicide give some warning signs such as verbalizing their feeling of committing suicide. Parents should not take it lightly but discuss this with their child and help him to understand that suicide is not a solution for a temporary problem. If you constantly support your child, he won't go into depression, and he will not have such as a suicidal tendency because suicide is an extreme form of depression.

Q. What should we do to improve memory power and concentration? Are there any programmes that help in doing so?

A. Yes, we strongly recommend programmes on how to improve the various learning modes and besides memory, comprehension, synthesis, analysis, etc. are important for all children.

Q. Do all students have examination stress?

A. No, all students are not susceptible to examination stress. Challenges are a part of the charm of life itself. Defining stress particular to examination system would be wrong. It is just a stepping-stone in life. Stress is not experienced by every child during the examination period. There are some who would be victims of phenomenal stress which may be physiological or psychological. We need to understand it from a holistic perspective including the physical, mental and social aspects.

Most of the children who go to counsellors or schoolteachers ask about how to manage time, how to prepare a particular chapter so that it does not accumulate for the last day. Many students report of irregular sleeping patterns, dietary patterns, mood swings, irritability, muscle aches and body aches. But these are not illnesses. Parents have to identify and learn to accept these changes as very nominal, normal changes for that period in life. These days, the media over-hypes the stress related to exams. Children have to accept the changing pattern of life in standard 10 or 12. A certain optimal amount of anxiety or stress is needed in life to perform better.

Q. How are schools helping students to accept these challenges?

A. I believe that chaos can be an opportunity. Schools these days are trying to distress pupils by creating an ethos that naturally brings forth this hype before the examinations. A lot of mechanisms are working in the school system today, such as the counsel mechanism, there is the school assembly where students can bring forth their problems; there are counselling sessions with social workers, with psychiatrists, etc. I think the basic idea is to perpetuate that exams are just one of the many things that happen during a student's life. The question of stress arises only when you are not in tune or socially contributing to the school environment. I believe in a phrase called NIMBI. NIMBI means, 'now I must be involved', which implys that now you should put away your cell phone and get to your books.

Q. I am not able to get proper sleep the day before my exam. Moreover, when I enter the examination hall, I don't feel confident that I have completed my course.

A. Firstly, don't ever think of taking any anti-anxiety or sedative pill that are commonly available at home.

Secondly, schoolchildren can do a simple breathing exercise – slow, deep, prolonged breathing just for about 4–5 minutes, 3–4 times a day. Doing this preferably before the exam can do wonders. Good amount of oxygen intake through our lungs will definitely promote a good memory.

Thirdly, don't try to cram up too much at the last minute. You are not supposed to revise the whole subject 12 hours prior to the exam. You should make bullet points much before the exam; you should go through the bullet points of every chapter one day before exam.

Fourthly, it is common that we tend to either over-eat or avoid eating at all during examinations, which is wrong. Spicy and salty food before the exams can lead to a lot of sluggishness in the examination timing. Green leafy vegetables, fruits, salads and pulses should be encouraged during examinations. Small meals prior to the exam help you to be more wakeful during the exam and also help in getting a restful sleep prior to the exam.

Lastly, communicating with family members is very important. Don't forget to sit across the dining table and share a few moments of togetherness with your family, discuss things which are not related to your exams. Repeat the same before leaving the house on the day of the exam. Don't think that you can go through the whole book in one minute while standing outside the examination hall. This can be disastrous, as the anxiety will make you feel amnesic about the whole subject. Rather, going to the examination hall with a blank mind is a good sign. It means that you know whatever you have internalized and you are going there without anticipating what is going to come in the exam. At least 5–6 hours of sleep before the exam is essential. Have your meal a little early in the evening, you can also have a midnight snack.

Q. **Do you think that parents accompanying their children to the examination hall add to the stress?**

A. Parents accompany their wards to centres because they need to be reassured that the child has reached the centre on time. It is not pampering of their wards at all. It is just the surety that the child has reached before time. I don't think we need to misunderstand the parents' concern regarding this.

Q. **What should be the role of parents during the exams?**

A. Parents' support is immensely important during a child's exams since they are the first and foremost source for the child's development. The parenting styles, the parenting patterns have taken a paradigm shift in the past 15–20 years, thanks to the globalization and the economic benefits. Undoubtedly, the emotional bonding has undergone a change that is inevitable. We are living in a rapidly changing world. Now expectations are very high; what is commonly seen as an ideal child syndrome, that is, can my child be an all rounder? Can he be perfect in everything? These conditions are pressurizing children subconsciously. Parents' expressions - verbal or non-verbal, their stress, their unfulfilled dreams can be perceived by the children. The expectations, comparisons between siblings, comparisons with the neighbour's child haunt the child during examinations. Your child needs you as a good communicator, as friend, as a comrade with whom he can communicate even the day before the exam. Little things, such as sitting on the dinning table together; watching television together, talking a walk with your child during the examination are helpful. Parents need to be a lot more aware of what's happening with their child and not impose their expectations and dreams on them.

Q. **What topics or areas should be included in the syllabus of educational psychology where prospective features and in-service features can be equipped to deal with situations which arise in schools?**

A. The topic of life skills programme should definitely be included in the curriculum. A very short course on what counselling is all about can also be included. Also, we should have a course on dialogue and expressing oneself. The CBSE has introduced a number of new courses, such as environmental education and they are in the process of introducing the life skill curriculum as well.

Q. **I am not able to maintain a proper routine prior to the examination because of my studies. I am not able to sleep on time, due to which I don't wake up on time. This affects my writing ability. What should I do?**

A. Firstly, as you are saying that you are not able to maintain a routine for yourself, you should consult a friend or a teacher. Secondly, you need to think about your weaker areas where you have to concentrate more. Thirdly, you should put up your datesheet on the wall and work backwards so that the last examination becomes the first one for you to study. Count how many hours you have every day and how much you can concentrate. Can you study for 2 hours at a stretch and then take a walk? Next you need to have a comfortable worktable with things that you like around you. Unless you are familiar with the place and enjoy sitting in the same place everyday, you will not be able to concentrate. If you like to walk around and study, do so. If you like to study with the music on, then convince your parents that you are comfortable about it.

Q. **I am not able to complete my syllabus, what should I do?**

A. You are not the only one who is not able to complete the syllabus. Normally, one prioritizes a number of questions. For example, instead of doing 30 questions, you take fewer topics say 5 questions and complete them with a greater degree of surety. Then prioritize another set of topics. Call up a teacher and get a time appointed to finish those topics. Please be happy and sure with what you have done already.

Q. **What exactly is stress? How can the parents and children know that they are going through it? What are its symptoms?**

A. We all agree that stress is inevitable, but our concern is largely focused on children who get into stress. Some of the stress indicators are lack of sleep, mood swings, indigestion, abdominal cramps, neckache and backache. The important part is that if these things are compounding and escalating, do feel comfortable to communicate or discuss them out. Contact the schoolteacher or a counsellor or even a psychologist so that you have one or two guided counselling sessions. This will help you to organize your 24-hour rhythm better. Medicines should be strictly avoided. Indigestion problems can he handled with antacids, or painkillers occasionally, unless prescribed by a doctor. The child may not express stress which builds up over a period of time. You need a special sense to detect stress from the child's voice and his day-to-day behaviour. You can understand better if you meet a counsellor.

Resources

American Academy of Pediatrics (AAP) – Parenting corner

http://www.aap.org/parents.html

The AAP website has information for professionals, as well as a parenting corner, with information on child and infant care, especially on thumb-sucking, selecting appropriate toys for children and safety tips.

CDC/National Center on Birth Defects and Developmental Disabilities (NCBDDD)

http://www.cdc.gov/ncbddd

The authoritative guide from CDC on child development provides tools for development disabilities, birth defects, ADHD, positive parenting tips, etc.

CDC/National Immunization Program

http://www.cdc.gov/nip/default.htm

A comprehensive guide for parents on childhood immunizations.

IndiaParenting

http://www.indiaparenting.com

This Indian website provides an interactive experience to parenting, with communities, interactive tools, message boards, etc., along with information on behavioural disorders and stammering.

KidsHealth

http://www.kidshealth.com

This website by The Nemours Foundation's Center for Children's Health

Media provides health information about children from before birth through adolescence, with separate sections for parents, kids and teens.

MedicineNet

http://www.medicinenet.com/healthy_kids/focus.htm

This website from WebMD focuses on the well-being of children from conception through adolescence, with all aspects of children's growth and development.

Medline Plus – Child development

http://www.nlm.nih.gov/medlineplus/childdevelopment.html

MedlinePlus brings together authoritative information on drugs, interactive tools for parents, latest health news, etc.

National Institute of Child Health and Human Development

http://www.nichd.nih.gov/

This National Institutes of Health's website provides information on developmental disabilities, including mental retardation, and the events that occur during pregnancy. It also conducts and supports research on all stages of human development, from preconception to adulthood.

Positive Parenting

http://www.parenting.org.uk/

Provide support to parents and those who work with them - they produce resources, training and the delivery of parenting support in the community.

Ministry of Child and Women Development – Food and Nutrition Board

http://wcd.nic.in/fnbweb.htm

This website from the Indian government provides sources of information on nutrition.

> If you have any similar questions which need an answer, please log on to our website (http://www.DoctorNDTV.com). We have more than 290 experts on our panel and their details are accessible at our website.